the HEART of HEALING

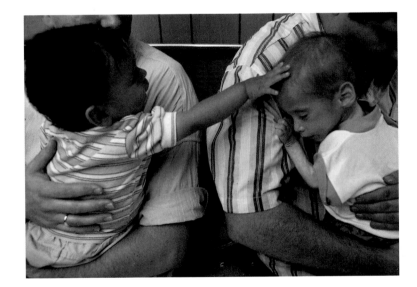

—INSTITUTE TEAM—
BRENDAN O'REGAN
CARYLE HIRSHBERG
NOLA LEWIS
BARBARA McNEILL
WINSTON FRANKLIN

the HEART *of* HEALING

THE INSTITUTE OF NOETIC SCIENCES WITH WILLIAM POOLE

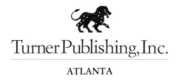

Turner Publishing, Inc.

ATLANTA

Published by Turner Publishing, Inc.

a subsidiary of Turner Broadcasting System, Inc.

1050 Techwood Drive, N.W.

Atlanta, Georgia 30318

Printed in the U.S.A.

First edition 10 9 8 7 6 5 4 3 2 1

ISBN 1-878685-44-9

Library of Congress Catalog Card Number: 93-60659

Distributed by Andrews and McMeel

A Universal Press Syndicate Company

4900 Main Street

Kansas City, Missouri 64112

Editor—*Katherine Buttler*
Copy Editor—*Erica Fox*
Editorial assistant—*Crawford Barnett*

Vice President Design/Production—*Michael J. Walsh*
Book Design—*Elaine Streithof*
Photo Researcher—*Marty Moore*
Photo Research Assistant—*Robin Luehrman*

Color separations/film preparation—*Hi-Tech Color, Smyrna, Georgia*
Jacket color separations/film preparation—*Graphics International, Atlanta, Georgia*
Printed and bound by R.R. Donnelley, Willard, Ohio

ACKNOWLEDGMENTS

This book, companion to the TBS television series *The Heart of Healing*, grew out of Brendan O'Regan's hope to increase public awareness of the field of mind-body health. In July 1987, as Vice-President for Research at the Institute of Noetic Sciences, Brendan presented his ideas to Institute directors. With the directors' support and in collaboration with television producer David Kennard, Brendan assembled the research data and financial resources that resulted in both the TV series and this book. Brendan died before this work was finished, but his vision inspired the rest of us to carry these projects to completion.

We are grateful for William Poole's conceptual ability as well as writing skills. He worked patiently over many months to help us organize volumes of research data and anecdotes into a coherent narrative. His sense of humor sustained us through innumerable rewrites and tight deadlines. Working with him is a pleasure.

The producers at Independent Communications Associates, Inc. (InCA) worked closely with Institute staff in coordinating the film treatment and book outline. Thanks, especially, to David Kennard and Joan Saffa.

Kathy Buttler, editor, Turner Publishing, Inc., was cooperative and gracious during the final months of book production, remaining calm and competent in the face of a looming deadline.

Beverly Rubik and Laura Franklin provided independent review and consultation on portions of the text. We thank them for their prompt and willing responses to our queries.

Finally we would like to thank the directors of the Institute of Noetic Sciences, Institute staff and colleagues, and 30,000 Institute members whose support made this book possible.

INSTITUTE OF NOETIC SCIENCES

CARYLE HIRSHBERG, NOLA LEWIS,
BARBARA MCNEILL, WINSTON FRANKLIN

TABLE OF CONTENTS

Title page spread: An integral part of the larger dimensions of healing is the love and support of others. These children with AIDS found a caring home with adoptive families.

Opposite page: Although Shin Teryama had less than three months to live, according to conventional doctors, he cured himself of kidney cancer with diet and faith in his body's ability to heal itself.

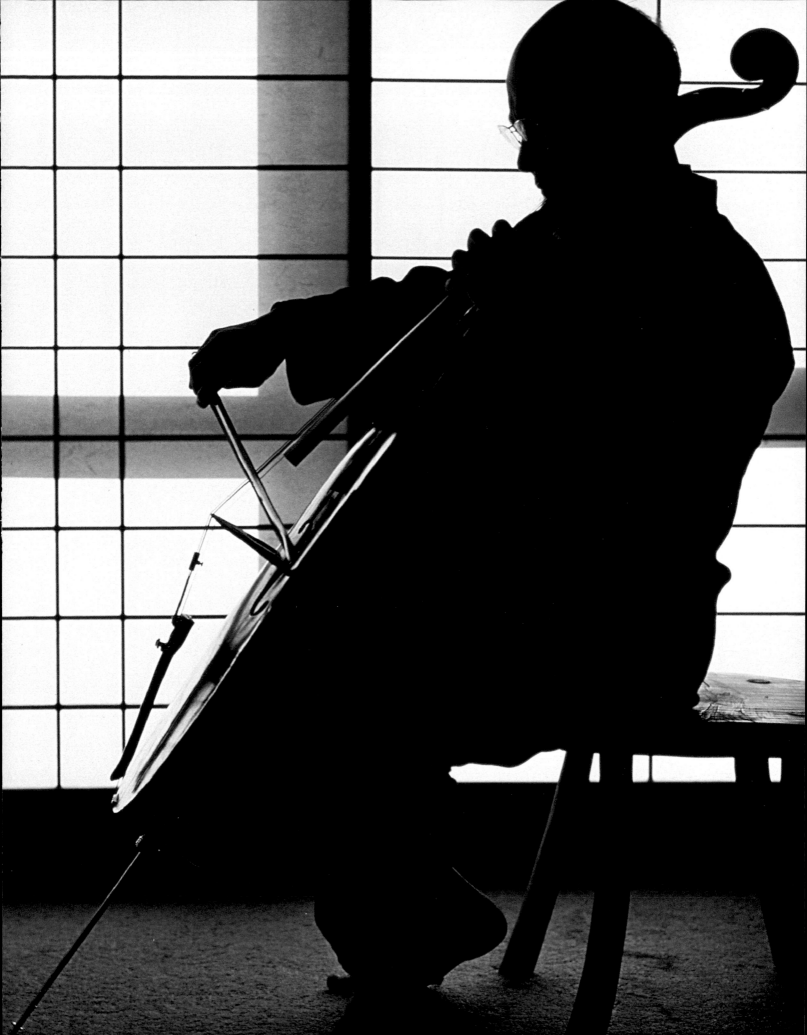

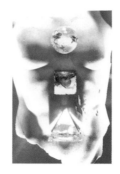

THE HEART OF HEALING

As Benjamin Franklin so aptly remarked, "God heals and the doctor takes the fee." Indeed, many illnesses seem to resolve themselves without extraordinary treatment. Over eons our bodies appear to have developed the ability to make routine repairs and even to defend us against illness or injury–both from within and without. Human beings are, in truth, self-healing creatures. If you nick your finger with a paring knife while preparing dinner, you can watch the healing start almost immediately. Specialized blood cells, called platelets, seal up the wound, stemming the flow of blood. White blood cells rush to the area to combat bacteria that might enter through the broken skin, and red blood cells arrive to nourish the healing tissue with oxygen. Over the next day or so, the small wound will quickly disappear. Likewise, a sprained ankle, a pulled shoulder, or a twisted knee will usually heal with a little rest. Broken bones will knit up as strong as ever and as straight as a surgeon can splint the pieces. And while decongestants can stanch the sniffles of a winter cold, it is your own healthy immune system that moves you back toward health. Each day, this system may prevent dozens of potential infections from developing.

Human self-healing is not invincible, of course. A person can bleed to death of a bad wound or die from

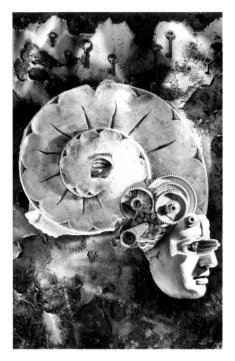

Opposite page:
Detail from
Reliquary
This page:
Wisdom
(Chapter One),
above. Detail
from *Epilogue*
(Chapter Two),
right.

a virulent infection. For reasons no one completely understands, our own cells can threaten us by raging out of control into a cancerous growth. When our self-healing system is overwhelmed, we call on medical science—although doctors are generally better at patching up injuries and subduing infections than at curing cancer or chronic diseases. What we call "health" requires more than a doctor's care. It results from an intricate balance between internal resources and outside conditions. Most of us know what we need to achieve this balance and maintain health: nutritious foods, adequate sleep and exercise, a clean and sanitary place to live, and an environment free of toxins and disease-causing microorganisms.

Most of us also understand instinctively that the mind has some role in health and healing. The "mind" is not only the brain, a bodily organ where much of the mind's work is accomplished, but also thought, emotion, will, perception, memory, imagination, and spirit. It is this mind that is credited with an important role in both curing and causing illnesses. The expression "It's all in your mind" is often used to explain why someone is ill. But increasing evidence shows that people can indeed "worry themselves sick"—that stress can be bad for the heart and anxiety can upset the stomach. Other people are said to be "too tough to die" or seem to survive on a "will to live," and many of us have noticed that we can sometimes control the timing of an illness—keeping ourselves going through academic exams or a big project at work, only to collapse when the hurdle is cleared.

During the last few decades doctors, psychologists, and biologists have been scrutinizing the mind's place in health and healing, and what they are learning rebuts the conception of the mind as somehow separate from the body. They are finding that the human is an indivisible whole; the mind is everywhere within the body, working to protect the health of the organism or perhaps allowing it to succumb to disease or death.

The mind influences body and health through the brain and central nervous system. The autonomic nervous system, which controls such things as blood flow to our extremities, is also linked to the mind, as you are reminded whenever you blush out of embarrassment. This system makes your palms sweat, speeds up your heart, and dumps acid into your stomach when you are under stress. For decades, doctors have understood how this system might also cause disease.

More recently, researchers have detailed subtle links

Turner Publishing commissioned artist Hans Neleman to create the conceptual art for the cover and chapter openers of *The Heart of Healing.* Raised in the Netherlands, Neleman is internationally respected for the unique use of light, texture, and symbolism in his still lifes.

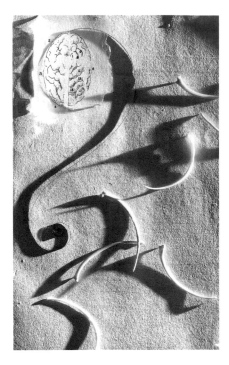

Detail from
Signifiers
(Chapter Three).

between the brain and the endocrine system, which releases body-controlling hormones, and the immune system, which guards against infection, cancer, and other illness. Psychoneuroimmunology (PNI)— a brand-new science with a hundred-dollar name— postulates that our psychological characteristics (our thoughts, feelings, and personality) are expressed through our neurological anatomy (our brain and nervous system) to affect our immunological defenses, and through them our health.

PNI anatomists and biochemists have discovered new neurological connections and more than fifty chemical messengers linking the brain to organs of the immune system. To this biological research have been added psychological studies showing how our personalities and coping styles, our feelings, our marriages and lifestyles, and our beliefs about the world and ourselves might influence our health through mind-body connections. Such research has swelled over the last few years—driven as much by public fascination as by any support from traditional institutional medicine. The public is also turning to alternative therapies based on a mind-body model. Increasingly, people are trying to maintain health and cure illness through meditation, hypnosis, group support, biofeedback, mental imaging, and simple positive thinking.

Many physicians have been skeptical about the role of mind in medicine, but this skepticism is gradually eroding in the face of evidence.

Detail from
Continuum
(Chapter Four).

Research is showing, for example, that breast cancer patients who receive group social support may live, on average, twice as long as those who do not. Other experiments have revealed that hypnosis can hasten the healing of burns, that laughter can increase immune function, and that diabetics can lower their need for insulin with deep relaxation techniques. Psychologists have sketched out personality types associated with heart disease, and studies linking psychological factors to illness and immune function now number in the thousands. This does not, of course, prove that humans can heal themselves of cancer or other disease. Nor does it prove that illness is "all in the head" or that we cause our own sicknesses. What the studies do suggest, however, is that feelings and emotions influence health, and that the body's healing system may be far more powerful and complex than we have dared imagine.

That's what this book is about: revealing and

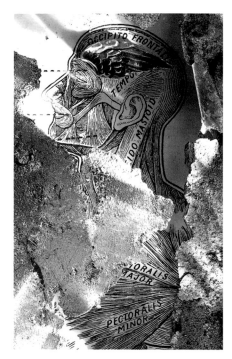

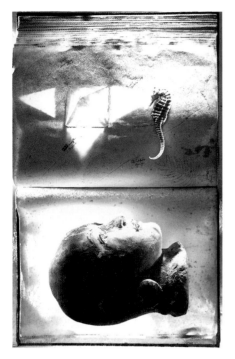

Detail from
Lifeline
(Chapter Five).

examining our remarkable system of self-repair which includes but goes far beyond the healing of wounds and the knitting of broken bones. For evidence of this system, we will look first at stories of those rare cancer patients who heal despite sentence of death. We will probe the role of expectation and belief in healing and ask why scientifically useless medications and treatments sometimes work.

While we look for evidence of a healing mind across the world's cultures, we will reveal the long association healing has had with faith, belief, spirit, family, the web of everyday life, and altered states of consciousness. We will trace Western medicine's narrow emphasis on the physical aspects of healing and wonder what may have been sacrificed for scientific "progress." After focusing on the immune system and the connections between healing, body, mind, and spirit, we will detail the growing body of evidence that thoughts, feelings, and attitudes can push us toward illness or toward health. Entering the mainstream are treatments for illness that now include hypnosis, meditation, visualization, and other self-healing techniques.

We will ask, finally, what this new knowledge about health and healing may mean in our lives: the effect of marriage on health and immune function; the health implications of childbirth, child rearing, career, maturity, and old age; and the growing evidence that community and family and friends are crucial to health. We will examine the impact of our society on health and will propose a re-examination of Western medicine's preoccupation with physical cures at the expense of the larger dimensions of healing.

Detail from
Phases
(Chapter Six).

In the beginning humans trusted what they observed about mind, body, spirit, and health—and what they observed was an inextricable interdependence. But in the nineteenth century, medicine became preoccupied with mechanisms and connections, with demonstrating how healing works. Much of the subsequent history of mind-body science is a history of the search for connections by researchers unwilling to dismiss our age-old instinct that the mind affects health.

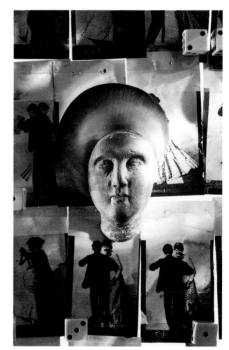

Psychoneuroimmunology and the other mind-body sciences are rediscovering the connections between feelings, thoughts, personality, and health. What we learn may ultimately help provoke a new revolution in medical science, placing the mind-body connection at the very heart of healing. If we are truly self-healing organisms, then humans may possess capacities and potentials about which we have only dared to dream.

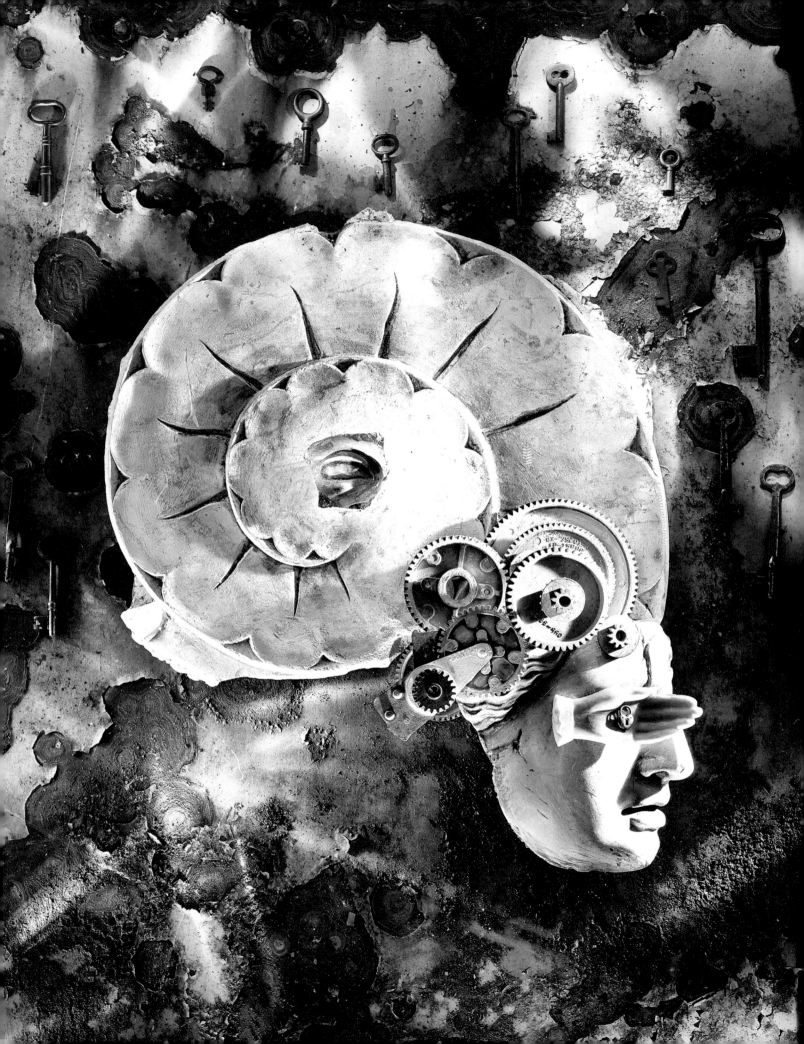

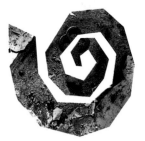

C H A P T E R   O N E

HEALING MYSTERIES

SIGNPOSTS OF A SELF-HEALING SYSTEM

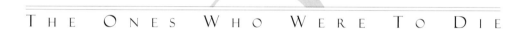

T H E   O N E S   W H O   W E R E   T O   D I E

N A JANUARY DAY IN 1983, a fifty-nine-year-old woman named Peggy McNeil departed the Valley Diagnostic Clinic in Harlingen, Texas, and went home to die. A few weeks earlier, McNeil had been sitting at her dining room table writing a letter when she reached her hand to her neck and felt a lump. Doctors at the clinic biopsied the lump—a swollen lymph node—and found it thick with large-cell carcinoma, a kind of cancer. An x-ray revealed a lurking shadow in Peggy McNeil's chest: a large tumor of the right lung from which the cancer had spread to the lymph node and might soon migrate throughout her body.

No operation was possible to remove such a tumor, Dr. Darvey Fuller told McNeil. With chemotherapy and radiation treatments, she might live a year or eighteen months, but the therapy would probably sap her energy and deny her valuable time. Without treatment, she would probably die in eight months. McNeil was clear on what she would do. "I had a lot to do and not much time for doing it," she would write later. "I had to stay in control as long as possible." Much to Dr. Fuller's surprise, Peggy McNeil did not die in eight months. She did not

> *"Miracles do not happen in contradiction of nature, but in contradiction of what we know about nature."* —SAINT AUGUSTINE (A.D. 354–430)

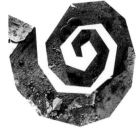

die in a year, or two years, or five. The lump in her neck disappeared. Nearly a decade later she is living with her husband in southern Texas, and her x-ray shows no tumor. When McNeil goes into the clinic these days, Dr. Fuller shakes his head in puzzlement and tells her that he doesn't know what she's doing but she shouldn't let up.

No one knows how many people like Peggy McNeil self-heal with little or no treatment from seemingly incurable cancer. Documented cases are certainly rare—many physicians work a lifetime without encountering one. But as rare as they are, such accounts offer our most dramatic evidence of the human ability to heal even from life-threatening illnesses.

Doctors use the terms *spontaneous regression* or *spontaneous remission* to describe an unexpected reversal of cancer or other disease. The word *spontaneous* implies that there is no cause for the unexpected improvements in the patient. But, of course, there is a cause, even if it is one we do not understand. *Regression* is used to describe the process in solid-tumor cancers, while *remission* may refer to these cancers as well as to cancers of the blood, such as leukemias and other diseases. To be considered spontaneous, a remission must occur without adequate treatment. Some spontaneous remissions are complete, last a lifetime, and are considered real cures. In other cases, the disease disappears for months or many years but returns later.

In the 1960s, two physicians named Tilden Everson and Warren Cole surveyed sixty years of American medical journals for examples of spontaneous remissions from cancer. Dr. Everson and Dr. Cole were tough reviewers. They excluded all cases of blood cancers—leukemias and lymphomas—because they can routinely go into remission. They also eliminated cases with any diagnostic uncertainty. Still, Everson and Cole found 176 cases in which a

cancer regressed without treatment or after treatment that, according to the doctors, generally should not have helped.

Recently, the Institute of Noetic Sciences has collected more than 3,500 accounts of spontaneous remission from 830 medical journals in more than twenty languages. Excerpts from these reports were published by the institute as *Spontaneous Remission— An Annotated Bibliography* in 1993. The earliest citation is from 1846—a report of spontaneous remission of a breast tumor—and the most recent reports date from the 1990s. In 15 percent of these cases, remission occurred without any therapeutic drugs or treatments. In other cases, remission followed partial or palliative surgeries or treatments that should not have produced cures. Spontaneous remission was reported from almost every disease, including every form of cancer.

One of the earliest carefully reported cases of spontaneous remission involved a thirty-one-year-old Baltimore woman who sought help for a lump and pain in her right breast. The breast was found to be cancerous and was surgically removed along with a nearby cancerous lymph node. After about a year of relative health, the woman developed pains in her back and leg, vision difficulties in her right eye, a new growth in her left breast, and a mass of tumor that rose directly from the center of her chest. She was prescribed morphine for pain and was soon confined to what her doctor assumed would be her deathbed.

The doctor's name was Sir William Osler, one of the fathers of modern American medicine. Dr. Osler sailed for England in June 1890, convinced that the woman would die before his return. But a year and a half later she met Osler at the train station. Her pain was gone, and the lump on her chest had vanished. "She had improved," Dr. Osler wrote, "in every way." Such cases suggested, he wrote, "that no condition, however desperate, is quite hopeless."

Lourdes and Other Miracles

One of the earliest stories of spontaneous remission dates from the thirteenth century, when a young Roman Catholic monk named Peregrine Laziosi was cured overnight of a leg tumor. Scheduled to undergo amputation of the leg the next day, Peregrine prayed for relief and dreamed that night that he was cured. The next morning the tumor was gone. Peregrine dedicated his life to the relief of suffering, until his death at the age of eighty in 1345. In 1726, Peregrine was canonized by the Catholic Church and became the patron saint of cancer sufferers. A pathologist named William Boyd once proposed that tumors that disappeared without treatment be designated Saint Peregrine Tumors.

Sudden healings like Peregrine Laziosi's, especially in a religious context, are sometimes thought of as miracles. No place is more associated with such miracles than the village of Lourdes, France. Near that town on February 11, 1858, a fourteen-year-old girl named Bernadette Soubirous was gathering firewood when she saw a white-clad vision of a woman who instructed her to dig in a sandy spot where Bernadette discovered a spring. Word soon spread that the woman had been the Virgin Mary and that the spring held the miraculous ability to cure the sick.

After a lengthy investigation, a special commission of the Catholic Church concluded that "the Immaculate Mary, Mother of God, did really appear to Bernadette Soubirous. . . . Our conviction is based on the testimony of Bernadette but more especially on the events which have occurred and which have no explanation save an intervention of God." More than four million pilgrims a year now visit Lourdes to worship or to bathe in the spring's miraculous waters.

If Everson and Cole were tough in reviewing claims of spontaneous remission, the medical authorities at Lourdes are tougher. Of the more than six thousand persons claiming cures since 1858, the church has officially recognized only sixty-five miracles. Pilgrims claiming cures are first examined by

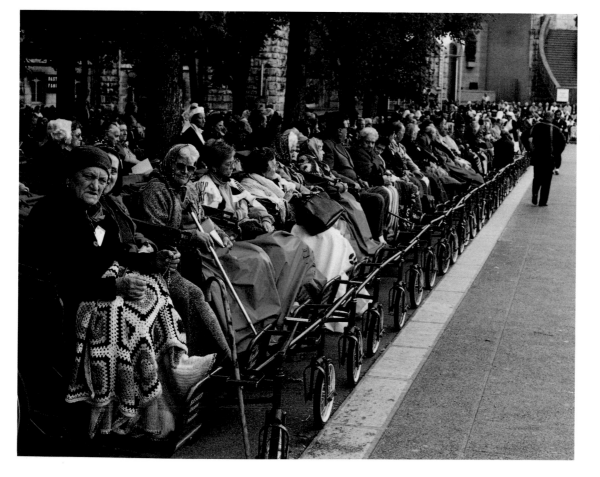

Each year more than five million people visit the Roman Catholic shrine in Lourdes, France, making it one of the most visited pilgrimage sites in the world.

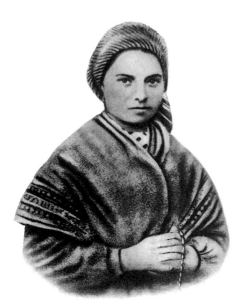

the Lourdes Medical Bureau, which opens a file, gathers data, and physically examines each claimant. Cases clearing that hurdle are then passed on to a twenty-five-member international committee of medical specialists, which conducts its own exhaustive investigation.

The medical examiners of Lourdes are looking for a special kind of spontaneous remission. In assessing a claim, the specialists must be satisfied that the diagnosis was accurate, the treatment was inadequate, and the disease was serious and in no way psychologically caused. Not only must the cure be considered complete, but it must contain an extra measure of inexplicability that might be evidence of a divine miracle. Much emphasis is put on the speed of the cure, since suddenness—as in the case of Saint Peregrine—is uncharacteristic of most remissions. By these criteria, a miracle may be seen as a spontaneous remission held to a higher standard.

Of course, the number and kinds of cures certified as miracles have changed over the years, reflecting medical progress. There were seven miraculous cures in the 1940s, ten in the 1950s, but only one in each decade of the 1960s and 1970s. Before the discovery of antibiotics in the mid-twentieth century, tuberculosis (TB) was a feared and widespread killer, and many early cures at Lourdes were from "incurable" cases of TB. Of the sixty-five cases certified as miracles, five, including two of the three most recent cases, have been cures of cancer.

Above: Bernadette Soubirous was fourteen years old when she reported her vision of the Virgin Mary near Lourdes, France. Below: Vittorio Micheli's cure from bone cancer is listed as the sixty-third of sixty-five officially recognized miraculous cures at Lourdes. Opposite page: Intensive prayer can contribute to an atmosphere of healing that leaves many Lourdes pilgrims feeling strengthened by their visit.

One such case is that of Vittorio Micheli, a member of the Italian Alpine Corps admitted to the military hospital of Verona in April 1962. The hospital record can only suggest what must have been a miserable and depressing dilemma for the twenty-two-year-old soldier. A sarcoma, a kind of cancer, had eaten into the bone at the top of his left leg and invaded the tissue around it, literally consuming the bone where the leg met the pelvis. There was little the doctors could do but immobilize his body in an enormous plaster cast. For more than a year Micheli lay in various hospitals. His appetite faltered, and his condition gradually deteriorated. When he announced that he wanted to go to Lourdes, the doctors exchanged his cast for a stronger one. With the plaster off, they examined his hip, which they found to be grossly deformed. They could feel no bones through the doughy mass of the tumor. They described the leg as "lifeless."

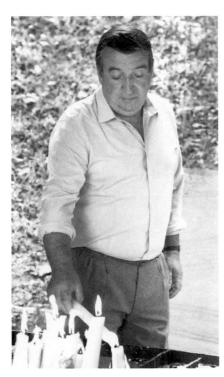

A few days later, Micheli was submerged in the water at Lourdes, cast and all. Immediately, he felt cured. He described a feeling of hunger and electricity passing through his body. On returning to the hospital, his appetite improved, and his pain subsided. He was up and walking within a month. At first there were no changes to his x-ray, but repeat films taken eight months later showed what doctors called "a remarkable reconstruction of the bony tissue of the pelvis."

It was this regrowth of the bone that seemed particularly inexplicable in Micheli's case, and led the medical examiners at Lourdes to label the case a miracle. Micheli left the hospital, walked with a cane for a while,

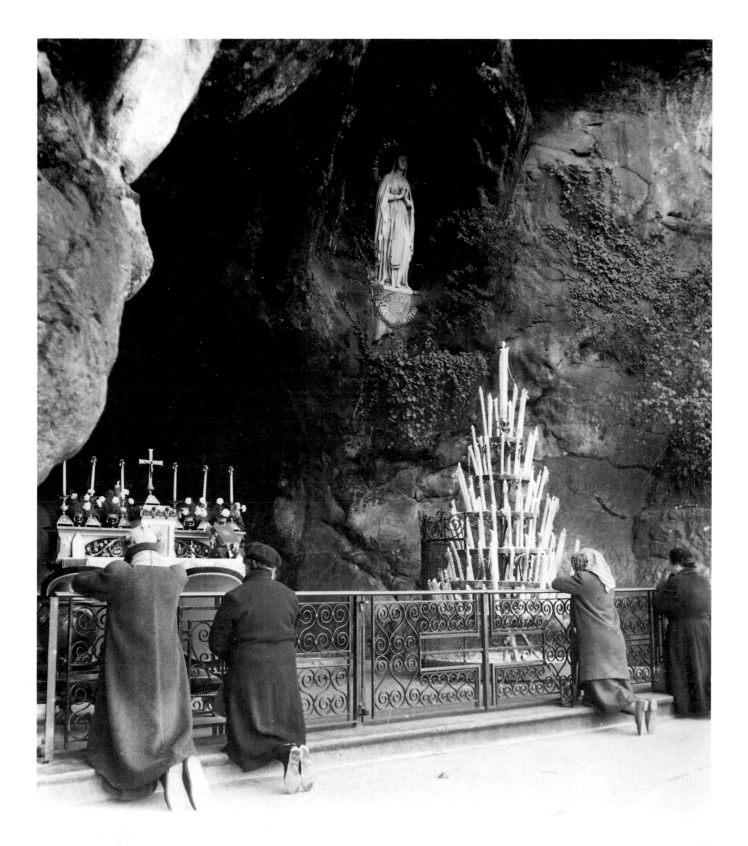

The first doctor to conduct an official examination of claims of miraculous cures at Lourdes was Baron de St. Maclou. In 1883, with the Catholic Church's approval, Dr. de St. Maclou began asking pilgrims who claimed to have been cured for medical certificates attesting to their having had specific organic diseases. He also invited other physicians to review these cases, thereby laying the groundwork for the Lourdes Medical Bureau, which today examines all pilgrims claiming to have been cured.

The rules used by the Catholic Church to determine that a cure is miraculous—at Lourdes or elsewhere—were first outlined by Cardinal Lambertini (later Pope Benedict XIV) in 1735. Nuances of interpretation have changed with the times, of course, but the rules remain basically the same. To be declared a miracle the cure must be of a disease that is serious and thought to be incurable. The disease must present a danger to life and must have a definite physical, not a psychological, cause. The disease must be proven to exist by biopsies, tests, and x-rays available for public examination. The disease must not be one from which patients sometimes recover on their own,

and the cure must not be attributable, to any degree, to medications or treatments the patient has received. Finally, the cure must be sudden, complete, inexplicable, and long-lasting— usually a minimum of three or four years.

If the doctors of the Medical Bureau believe a cure may be inexplicable, they invite the pilgrim to return for a follow-up examination. Meanwhile, the doctors gather data on the case, including pertinent tests and x-rays. If the pilgrim's file is kept open—because the doctors still believe a cure may be inexplicable—the patient is asked to return for at least two more annual examinations.

At one time, the Medical Bureau had the final word in authenticating inexplicable cures. Since 1947, however, cases that pass the bureau's scrutiny have been passed on to the International Medical Committee of Lourdes, which is composed of about two dozen medical specialists from across Europe. The committee usually meets once a year. If a case passes an initial evaluation, it is assigned to one or two committee members, who usually examine the patient, peruse records, interview doctors, and prepare a full report. The report is then discussed by the committee at length under

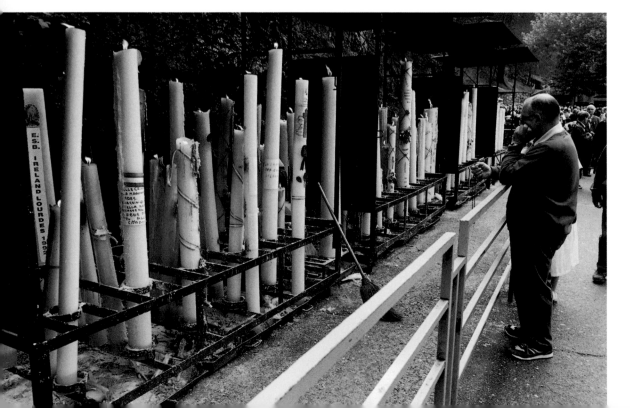

This page: The Massabielle Grotto. Opposite page: The Chapel of St. Bernadette.

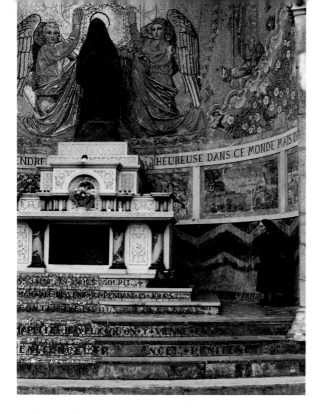

eighteen headings designed to satisfy Cardinal Lambertini's criteria. Committee members vote on each heading, with a simple majority being necessary for approval. The process is still not over, since attributing a cure to God is a religious, not a medical, assertion. The final determination is made by the bishop of the patient's diocese, who may appoint a church commission with its own medical advisers.

Not surprisingly, the number of cures meeting Cardinal Lambertini's ancient criteria has dropped as medical science has grown more sophisticated and treatment more widespread. Most people now claiming relief from a serious disease have undergone some kind of treatment, eliminating the cures from consideration as miracles.

The International Medical Committee last declared a cure a miracle in 1982, although thousands of people *feel* they have been cured at Lourdes, even if they do not meet the formal criteria. Thousands more gain inspiration, strength, spiritual succor, and a renewed perspective on their suffering after making a pilgrimage. This may help explain why Lourdes is one of the most popular pilgrimage sites in the world—more popular than Jerusalem, Mecca, or Rome. Such an atmosphere of healing is surely, in its own way, miraculous.

and was fitted with a special shoe to compensate for the difference in the length of his legs. Later he would hike in the mountains, play sports, and return to work.

Whether you view Micheli's cure as a divine miracle or an extreme example of spontaneous remission will depend in part on the specifics of your faith. "Believers and unbelievers must let the facts speak for themselves," wrote Michel-Marie Salmon, surgeon in chief of the Academy of Surgery of France, in summarizing the Micheli case for the Lourdes committee of specialists. They should do this, he wrote, "so that the believer does not see extraordinary cures everywhere . . . and the unbeliever does not take refuge in denial or skepticism."

What Causes Spontaneous Remission?
Why should some cancers and other diseases inexplicably improve on their own? Physicians have little idea, in part because the subject has not been studied much. There is no current textbook on spontaneous remission, no journal devoted to it, no listing for "spontaneous remission" in the most common medical indices—despite the valuable information these cases might hold. As Dr. Charles Mayo wrote in 1963, "To understand the basis of such cures would be to gain fundamental knowledge about the control of malignant growths and the host-tumor relationship."

Mayo, a surgeon at Minnesota's Mayo Clinic, had his own reason for being curious. In May 1950, he had operated on a sixty-three-year-old woman suffering from cancer of the colon, which had spread to nearby lymph nodes and both lobes of her liver. Mayo reasonably believed that the woman was doomed. He considered the surgery palliative—that it would relieve, at least temporarily, the patient's bloody diarrhea.

The woman was discharged without ever being told she had cancer—which would be unlikely to happen today. Mayo told the woman's family that she probably would live eight or nine months. Twelve years later, the clinic received a letter from the woman's son. "Since five years without recurrence of a cancer is considered a cure," he wrote, "could it be that this was a case of self-cure, about which I have

THE HEART   19

OF HEALING

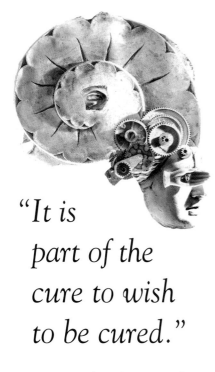

"It is
part of the
cure to wish
to be cured."

—SENECA (3 B.C.–A.D. 65)

read several reports?" Mayo brought the woman into the hospital. Her physical examination, her x-ray examination, her blood count, and her blood chemistry revealed no evidence of cancer. On the reason for the cure, Mayo wrote, "one can only speculate."

Doctors do have some clues to the causes of spontaneous remissions. Some cancers seem more likely to regress than others. Melanomas— cancers of melanin-producing skin cells—are one such cancer, as are cancers of the kidney, certain cancers of the lymph system, and choriosarcoma, a tumor of the female reproductive system. Neuroblastoma, a cancer arising in the nerve cells of fetuses and infants, comes in two forms, one of which remits up to 80 percent of the time. Some doctors do not even treat this form of neuroblastoma except with simple surgery. Typically, in this case, cancer cells remain in evidence, but the tumor disappears and never comes back.

A variety of medical events have been associated with remissions. Remissions sometimes follow palliative or partial surgeries, as with Dr. Mayo's patient. They also seem to follow limited treatments of radiation, biopsy procedures, or high fevers. Any of these events may provoke changes in body chemistry or immune function that reverse the development of the tumor.

Mental processes may also trigger the chemical and immune changes that encourage remission. Even a decade ago such a proposal would have seemed preposterous. But as we shall see in the following chapters, researchers are gathering evidence that the mind plays an essential role in physical processes. Exactly what effect mental processes might have in curing diseases is not known.

A few researchers have tried to demonstrate an association between psychological processes and cases of remission, usually by looking for common psychological characteristics or events. They have found that a dramatic life change is sometimes a theme in these cases. Charles Weinstock, a psychiatrist and professor at the Albert Einstein College of Medicine in New York, studied eighteen consecutive cases of spontaneous remission from his practice and found they were all preceded by a "favorable psycho-social change" within one to three weeks. "The changes," Weinstock wrote, "ranged from religious conversion, to reconciliation with a long-hated mother, to a sudden marriage, and the death of a long-hated husband." Similarly, Dr. Yujiro Ikemi, of the Department of Psychosomatic Medicine at Kyushu University in Japan, discovered life changes in five Japanese cases that came to his attention. This "dramatic change of an outlook on life . . . seemed to have led to the full activation of their innate self-recuperative potentials."

In a slightly more systematic study, Dr. Marco de Vries, of Erasmus University in the Netherlands, compared six patients who had self-cured of cancer with six patients who eventually died of the disease. In structured interviews, de Vries and his colleagues evaluated each patient in a number of areas, including awareness and beliefs about diagnosis,

Shin Terayamo stopped playing the cello after being diagnosed with metastic kidney cancer. He was too tired and sick. Then, after advice from a friend who was a holistic medical counselor, Terayamo changed his diet and became a participant in his own healing. Soon he was recovering from his disease and was playing his cello again.

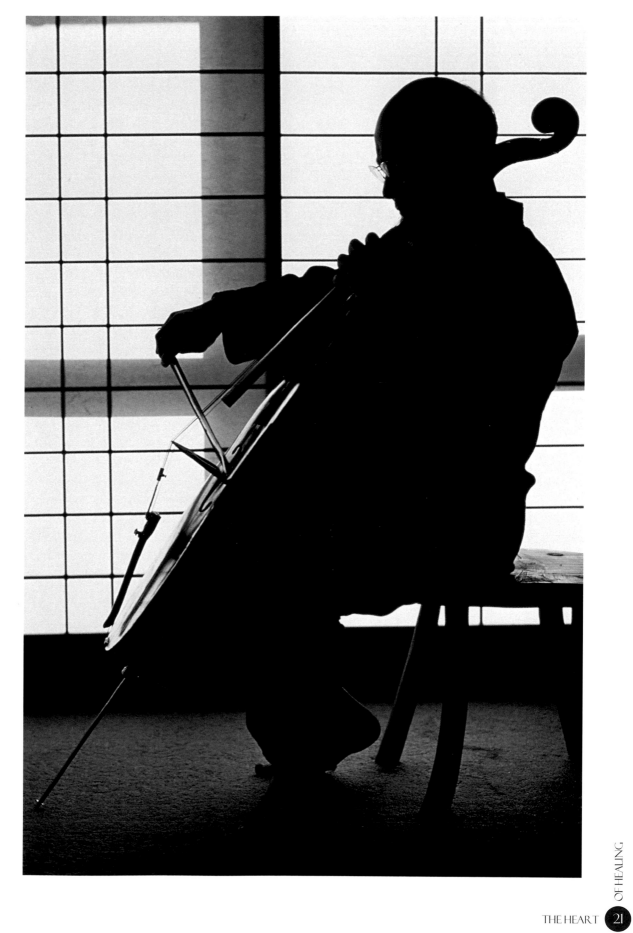

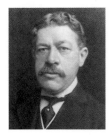

No one knows exactly why some people unexpectedly recover from cancer or other life-threatening diseases. But doctors have noticed that some people seem to recover in a predictable pattern following other medical events. One significant discovery came in 1891, after a young New York surgeon named William B. Coley (above) lost his first patient to widespread sarcoma, a soft-tissue cancer. Dr. Coley was upset enough about the patient's death to research similar cases in the files at New York Hospital. In medical records dating back more than a century, he began to notice case after case in which recovery from sarcoma followed a serious streptococcal infection known as erysipelas.

Could it be that the infection and fever were prompting the body to attack the tumor? Coley tested the idea by injecting bacteria directly into the tumors of sarcoma patients. After some experimentation, he eventually developed a mixture of heat-killed bacteria that became known to the world as Coley's toxins. About an hour after an injection, the patient would be gripped by shaking and chills followed by a raging fever. These symptoms usually subsided in less than twenty-four hours—just in time for many of the patients to receive the treatment again. The first patient treated with Coley's toxins, a nineteen-year-old boy with sarcoma of the pelvis, endured the injections every day or so for almost four months. And although he received no other medicine, treatment, or surgery, in time he recovered completely.

Coley's toxins were eventually injected into hundreds of patients for whom no other therapy was available. The treatments seemed most potent against sarcoma: one study found that 50 percent of the patients survived five years or more (compared to one contemporary report of less than 30 percent survival from such tumors). In the same study, 38 percent of the patients suffering from lymph node cancers survived for five years. The few breast cancer patients Dr. Coley treated did not do as well. The severity of the fever and associated chills seemed an important element in the treatment. Patients suffering the highest fevers—between 102 and 105 degrees—were more than twice as likely to benefit from the injections. This seemed to suggest that in some way the body's natural reaction to the infection destroyed the tumor.

After Coley's death in 1936, interest in his theories and treatments gradually declined, perhaps because of the introduction of chemotherapy and radiation as new therapies for cancer. But Coley's daughter, Helen Coley Nauts, took up her father's work. She collected more than fifty thousand articles on Coley's toxins and associated subjects and authored scholarly papers and went on to found the Cancer Research Institute in New York, which distributes more than $6 million a year for innovative cancer research.

In 1976, Nauts asked Dr. Lloyd Olds, of the Memorial Sloan Kettering Cancer Center in New York, to study Coley's toxins using rapidly evolving laboratory techniques. In response, Olds asked Nauts if she could come up with one hundred documented cases in which the toxins had produced remission. When Nauts returned with one thousand cases, Olds agreed to do the work. Olds and his associates implanted tumors into mice and injected those tumors with Coley's toxins. Eventually, they isolated a cancer-attacking chemical from the blood of the mice that they named tumor necrosis factor. This chemical, which has since been genetically cloned and used in patients in clinical trials, is produced by the immune system, apparently in reaction to infection and fevers. This and similar work is leading to a new class of cancer treatments based on the immune system's response to tumors. One hundred years after William Coley first noticed that some cancers get better after infections, he is recognized by many as the first cancer immunologist.

trust in medical procedures and doctors, hopelessness and depression, autonomy, social support systems, and marked changes in daily activity or outlook on life. On average, the scientists found, patients who remitted from cancer had been less depressed and more autonomous than those who died of their disease. They had been less trusting of medical opinion and diagnosis and benefited from more solid support systems.

All the patients had experienced what de Vries called "a more or less radical existential shift" for the better. One patient, a female student, was able to form a stable relationship with a man, which she had resisted before her illness. Another patient reported becoming "much more gentle with other people. . . .

I enjoyed the time I had been given to turn into myself, attend to what I am essentially doing, what I am going to make of my life."

Depression, optimism, autonomy, social support, positive life changes: We are gradually learning how to measure the effect of all of these factors on health. But we are a long way from understanding what part, if any, they play in the unexpected cure of deadly disease. We all know of optimistic and autonomous people who enjoyed loving and supportive families and exciting and rewarding work yet died of cancer. For now, self-healing of cancer and other diseases must be considered a great wonder and our most extreme evidence of how much we have yet to learn about human healing.

THE MYSTERIOUS PLACEBO

If there is a single patient renowned in the annals of mind-body medicine, it is the unfortunate Mr. Wright, who suffered from cancer of the lymph nodes in the mid-1950s. Mr. Wright (a pseudonym) was a patient of Dr. Philip West and of Dr. Bruno Klopfer, a psychiatrist who later made the case famous by reporting on it in the *Journal of Projective Techniques and Personality Assessment*.

Wright was near death when he learned that Krebiozen, a new, highly touted cancer drug, would soon be available for trial. Tumors the size of oranges had swollen in Wright's neck, under his arms, and in his groin, chest, and abdomen. He burned with fever and required oxygen. His physicians believed he was "in a terminal state, untreatable, other than to give him sedatives to ease him on his way."

Wright was too sick to qualify for the experimental drug, but he begged his doctors to give it to him. He received his first dose of Krebiozen on a Friday and became so sick that Dr. West believed that this first dose might be the last. But on Monday morning West found the patient "walking around the ward, chatting happily with the nurses, and spreading his message of good cheer to anyone who would listen. . . . The tumor masses had melted away like snowballs on a hot stove, and in only these few days, they were half their original size." When Wright's startled doctors finally

discharged him from the hospital ten days later, the disease had all but vanished.

A fairy tale version of the story would end here, but Wright's was far from over. Soon there was troubling news about Krebiozen. Very few patients improved on the drug, and newspapers were announcing that the "wonder drug" might be a flop. Wright followed this publicity grimly, and, after two months of good health, gradually relapsed to his moribund state.

Dr. West decided to conduct an experiment. He reassured Wright that the newspapers were wrong, that Krebiozen was as promising as ever, and that the relapse was due only to a decline in the drug's potency. Deliberately playing on his patient's optimism, West promised that a shipment of "super-refined, double-strength" Krebiozen was on the way. "By delaying a couple of days before the 'shipment' arrived," West wrote, "his anticipation of salvation had reached a tremendous pitch. When I announced that the new series of injections were about to begin, he was almost ecstatic and his faith was very strong."

Wright's second recovery was even more dramatic than the first—although this time he was injected with nothing more than sterile water. Once again the tumors diminished, and soon the patient was "the picture of health." And so he remained until the

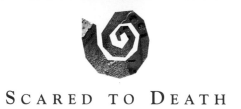

SCARED TO DEATH

How powerful is the action of belief on the human body? This Biami tribesman of Papua, New Guinea, lay down to die simply because he believed that sorcery had been worked on him. And he did die, within a single day, for reasons science cannot fully explain.

Scientists sometimes call such deaths "voodoo deaths"—a reference to the magical religion of voodoo, which arose in West Africa and was brought to the Americas with slavery. Adherents of voodoo and similar widespread religions believe that spirits may promote good or evil and that a person may be blessed or cursed through sorcery. Voodoo deaths do not result from heart attacks or other understood disease. Some deaths are sudden, and may result from a kind of nervous collapse in the face of overwhelming fright. As in so many mind-body mysteries, belief seems to be the key.

Renowned Harvard physiologist Walter Cannon, who investigated voodoo deaths in the 1940s, put it this way: "The force that really killed . . . was the fatal power of the imagination working through unmitigated terror."

Cannon reported on a case from North Queensland, Australia. Rob, a young native working with a local missionary, had been cursed by having a bone pointed at him by a powerful sorcerer named Nebo, whose people were being cared for by the mission. A visiting physician examined Rob and found him to have "no fever, no complaint of pain, no symptoms or signs of disease." Yet the young man was in obvious distress and weakening quickly. The visiting physician and the missionary went to Nebo with an ultimatum: If anything happened to Rob, Nebo's people would receive no more food and would have to leave the mission. "At

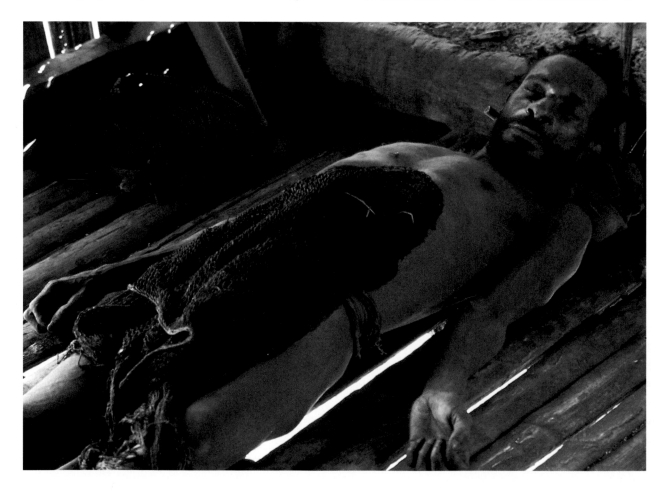

once, Nebo agreed to go with them to see Rob," Cannon wrote. "He leaned over Rob's bed and told the sick man it was all a mistake, a mere joke." Rob's relief was almost instantaneous. He was entirely well and back at work that evening.

Another less happy case was reported in the *American Journal of Psychiatry* in 1977 by Kenneth Golden, a former Peace Corps volunteer who had lived and worked in West Africa. Golden's native landlady, a prosperous woman in her thirties, had suffered from severe and mysterious stomach pains and had undergone three exploratory surgeries without discovery of the cause. Gradually, the woman lost weight and died. No funeral was held—a dramatic breach of custom—and when asked why, the villagers stated that the woman had died of a curse because she had been an adulteress. This story highlights the role of the community in voodoo deaths. Because family and neighbors believe in the curse, they may ostracize the victim. Researchers have suggested that some voodoo deaths are culturally sanctioned ritual suicides in which the community plays a key role. Thus, the cause of these deaths is not only terror and hopelessness, but also loneliness and isolation. The victim may remain isolated until the inevitability of death is accepted.

Voodoo deaths are an example of a much larger phenomenon—a failure of the will to survive. Modern animal research has shown that helplessness and despair can lead to the abandonment of survival-oriented behaviors. Cambodian tribesmen relocated to America after the Vietnam War developed a mysterious and fatal wasting sickness, apparently caused by hopelessness, isolation, futility, and despair.

Although the precise biological mechanisms of voodoo death are not known, it is clear that a powerful relationship exists between belief and survival. The placebo response is a two-edged sword: It not only cures but kills.

American Medical Association came forward with a formal announcement: "Nationwide tests show Krebiozen to be a worthless drug for the treatment of cancer." Within days, a dejected Wright checked into a hospital and quickly died.

The Mind's Medicine
Krebiozen is on a long list of drugs and treatments discredited by scientific medicine. At one time healers' remedies have included crushed spiders, eunuch fat, unicorn horn, lizard's blood, scrapings from the skull of a hanged criminal, and powdered mummy. What is most interesting about these discredited pills and potions, however, is not that they were not effective, but that, like Krebiozen, they *were* effective for some patients some of the time. If it was not the drugs that made these patients better, what was it? Perhaps the power of their own minds.

Western medicine calls substances that have a suggestive effect *placebos*, from the Latin word *placere*, meaning "to please." A placebo is, according to one early writer, "any medication adopted more to please than to benefit the patient." The definition betrays a persistent prejudice. Doctors and the federal government have long required any new drug to prove its effectiveness in tests against "sugar pills" or similar placebos. By focusing on the effectiveness of the test drug—on the healing from the outside— doctors have largely ignored those patients who improve on the placebo alone.

For these patients, the healing comes from the inside and the placebo is merely a prompt. For a landmark 1955 study, Harvard physician Henry Beecher reviewed fifteen double-blind studies in which patients were given placebos to treat headache, seasickness, anxiety, pain, or the common cold. Overall, 35 percent of the subjects were relieved of their complaints. Yet we still think of this inner-controlled healing as somehow different from "real medicine."

Spontaneous remissions offer rare but radical proof of the human ability to self-heal, but evidence of self-healing from placebos is both common and widespread. Studies have suggested that perhaps a third of the drugs prescribed in the United States may work primarily through the placebo effect. Healers

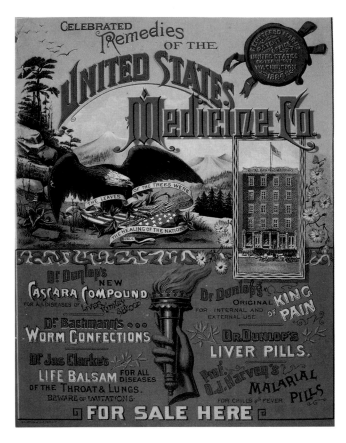

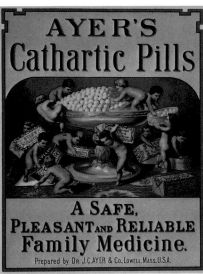

Throughout history, most medicines seemed to work for at least some patients—perhaps in part because of the placebo effect.

and philosophers in every culture across the breadth of human history have recognized that a patient's expectation and belief about treatment can influence the outcome of treatment. As the Roman philosopher Seneca wrote, "It is part of the cure to wish to be cured." In the book *Anatomy of an Illness*, in which American journalist Norman Cousins recounts his own unexpected recovery from life-threatening disease, he calls the placebo effect "the chemistry of the will to live."

Drugs are not the only placebos. The effectiveness of medical treatments and even surgery may depend at least in part on the placebo effect. In the late 1950s, American surgeons developed an operation to relieve heart pain, known as angina pectoris. Anginal pain occurs when not enough blood reaches the heart muscle, so the surgeons attempted to detour blood to the heart by tying off a nearby artery. A debate soon arose about the value of these operations. Some surgeons were enthusiastic and reported pain relief in as many as 75 percent of their cases. More skeptical surgeons reported lower rates of success.

What happened next could not happen today, with the emphasis on patients' rights and informed consent for all procedures. Several surgeons decided to test the angina operation by performing placebo surgeries in which they cut open their patients and then closed them back up again without tying off the artery. These patients experienced everything the medical system could offer—the attention of their doctors, the drama of preparing for surgery, the surgical incision, nurturance during recovery, and the expectation that the new and widely hailed treatment would improve their condition—except the treatment itself. The doctors found that the phony surgeries proved no less beneficial to patients than the real thing. In one study, *more* patients who'd undergone the sham operation reported relief. Placebo surgery reduced the patients' use of nitroglycerin, the most common pain reliever for angina. It also increased patients' capacity for exercise and the amount they could work.

The Biology of Belief

Placebo research has led to a new appreciation of the role of belief and expectation in healing. The effectiveness of even the most proven drugs may be increased by what has been called the "placebo halo"—the patient's expectation that the drugs will help. Nurses notice that even the way a medication is given can affect a patient's expectations about its results. Patients assume an injection is "stronger medicine" than a pill and capsules are more potent than tablets.

Doctors long ago recognized that the excitement generated about any new medication seemed to increase its efficacy—presumably because physicians communicated this excitement to their patients. Similarly, one recent study revealed that treatments and drugs worked particularly well if prescribed by the doctors who'd introduced them and therefore had particular faith in their success. Such knowledge is enshrined in an old medical adage: "Treat as many patients as possible with the new drugs, while they still have the power to heal." The force of a doctor's personality and ability to express concern for patients, the white coat and stethoscope, and the shiny high-tech gear of the modern hospital may all affect a patient's attitude toward therapy, and so influence the result.

Rituals also may help form our attitudes about healing, and so influence whether or not we heal. As we discuss in the next chapter, healing is associated with elaborate rituals in many cultures and settings. Trips to the doctor's office, the routine of hospital admission, and the daily regimen of pills and treatments contribute to our expectation that we will be healed. Likewise, might not at least part of the healing evidenced at Lourdes occur because the pilgrimage, with its attendant planning and ceremony, is so emotionally charged?

Studies have shown that patients who expect positive results from medical treatments are more likely to have them. In one study, patients awaiting eye surgery were given a questionnaire to measure their attitudes toward the operation. Those whose scores indicated the highest acceptance of the procedure healed more rapidly following surgery, as judged by an ophthalmologist with no knowledge of the test scores. Optimism and trust were key attitudes in those who healed most quickly. "The person seeking to help the slow healer . . . should focus primarily on what variables enhance or destroy the

Research has long shown that placebos may work as well as if the patient had taken actual medicine. Key to this effectiveness seems to be the patient's belief in the doctor and the medical system.

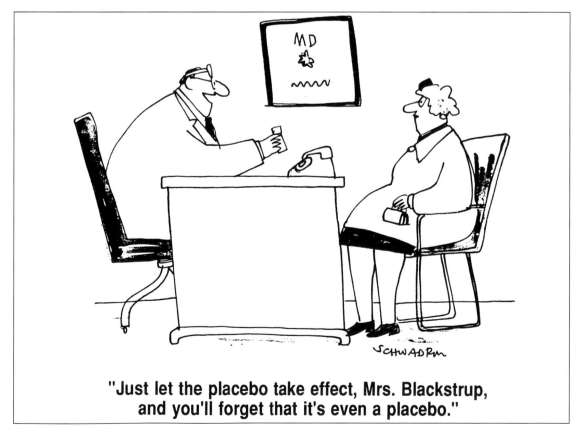

"Just let the placebo take effect, Mrs. Blackstrup, and you'll forget that it's even a placebo."

patient's attitude of expectant faith," the researchers concluded.

In the 1950s, German physician Hans Rehder reported how expectant faith helped three of his slow-healing patients. The patients—all women—were suffering from different diseases. One was disabled by a chronically inflamed gallbladder, the second was mysteriously wasting away from abdominal surgery, and the third suffered from a swollen abdomen and widespread cancer of the uterus. After all conventional treatment had failed, the doctor conceived an experiment for the three women. First he approached a local spiritual healer, who claimed to be able to project his healing powers at a distance. Initially, the women were not told about the healer, and his treatments seemed to have no effects. Then the doctor, with much fanfare, told the women of the healer and his powers. A date and time were set for a "distant" healing, and the women were encouraged to anticipate a wonderful change.

In fact, the healer made no effort to project his powers on the women that day. But within days the women began to heal. The first patient's chronic gallbladder inflammation cleared and remained in remission for many years. After months of weight loss, the second patient gained thirty pounds and was discharged from the hospital, essentially cured. The third patient shed fluid from her swollen belly, and, although she ultimately died of her disease, she lived her last few months at home with relative strength and comfort. Each healing seemed to extend from the anticipation of healing itself.

The biology of belief does not always have positive results, of course. Patients given placebo drugs have reported a wide range of side effects—including drowsiness, nausea, diarrhea, sleep disturbance, and skin rashes—apparently because they believed such side effects might occur. In 1983, the *World Journal of Surgery* reported a large study on the effectiveness of various chemotherapies for certain types of cancer. As in all studies of this kind, some patients received placebos. The study also reported on side effects, including hair loss, which is a common and expected result of chemotherapy. Buried in the data was the startling revelation that fully 30 percent of the patients given the placebo had lost their hair.

How Some Placebos May Work

Not long ago placebo effects were thought to be largely subjective. It was argued that patients who responded to placebos did not really get better, but simply felt better. A placebo was thought to be a kind of psychological trick. In fact, placebo drugs and treatments have demonstrated widespread physical effects, including coughs, skin rashes, and alterations in reaction time, grip strength, pulse rate, blood pressure, and stomach action. Noting such effects is one thing, but learning exactly how a placebo may work is another. In 1978, a single study forever changed the debate about how placebos may work, at least in the specific area of pain relief. By the late 1970s, researchers were beginning to understand that the body produces powerful pain relievers similar in chemical structure to morphine and other narcotic drugs. Such chemicals—called endorphins—are released in times of stress and block specific pain receptors in the brain. With this knowledge, researchers wondered whether expectation and belief might also prompt the release of endorphins and explain why placebo drugs worked for pain.

The 1978 study involved patients at a San Francisco clinic who had been experiencing severe dental pain after having surgery to remove impacted wisdom teeth. In a randomized trial, almost 40 percent of the patients who received placebos experienced significant pain relief—which came as little surprise to the researchers. A little while later, half those patients also received a dose of naloxone, a drug that blocks the effects of endorphins at the pain-receptor sites. Almost immediately, they started to complain of pain again. This seemed to suggest that the placebo had stimulated the body's internal pain relief system.

It is now clear that this conclusion may have been oversimplified. Studies have since suggested that pain relief from placebos is far more complex. But the finding that there is a link between placebos and endorphins was a pioneering discovery in the science that would become psychoneuroimmunology. As we shall see in Chapter Three, endorphins and their chemical cousins are now thought to be part of an ever-elaborating network linking thoughts, feelings, beliefs, and expectations to health.

THE HEALING POWER OF TRANCE

In March 1784, King Louis XVI of France appointed a royal commission to investigate the healing techniques of an expatriate Viennese physician named Franz Anton Mesmer. To head the commission, he chose seventy-eight-year-old Benjamin Franklin, U.S. ambassador to France. As a foreigner, Franklin may have seemed an unusual choice, but his stature as a scientist was unchallenged, and he enjoyed immense popularity with the French people. In addition to Franklin and others, the commission included Dr. Antoine-Laurent Lavoisier, who would be called the father of modern chemistry, and physician Joseph-Ignace Guillotin, who would go on to invent the automatic decapitation device that bears his name and in which King Louis himself would eventually lose his head.

For the time being, however, it was Mesmer who had Louis in a fix. Mesmer's extravagant claims and growing popularity had provoked suspicion and envy in the Parisian medical establishment. Furthermore, Mesmer was the toast of Paris—a witty, charming, dramatic man who had attracted and satisfied many prominent patients, including the king's own wife, Marie Antoinette. Something Mesmer was doing seemed to be healing them, as plenty of citizens were willing to attest.

Mesmer believed in what he called "animal magnetism," a basic life force present in the body in the form of a vital fluid. The depletion of this liquid could lead to assorted mental and physical diseases, Mesmer concluded. Its restoration, through "magnetic treatments," could restore bodily balance and health. Such theories ran counter to eighteenth-century rationalist science, particularly medicine, which was trying to establish itself as firmly based on measurement and experimentation. To most French doctors, Mesmer's belief in a universal magnetic life force seemed a throwback to medieval superstition.

The goal of Mesmer's treatments was to produce a kind of fit or trance in the patient by transferring magnetism from either Mesmer or his magnetized paraphernalia. After this, Mesmer believed, a healthy balance of magnetic fluid would be restored. Most of Mesmer's patients were women, to whom he would sit very close, making "passes" with his hands over the affected parts of their bodies. For group treatments, he would appear in a silk lilac-colored robe, carrying a metal "magnetic" rod. His patients—often roped together—sat grasping similar metal rods protruding from an oak bucket filled with bottles of special "magnetized" water. Mesmer would lead the group in chanting and in songs and prompt the participants to circle the bucket in a kind of dance. The royal commission investigating Mesmer reported that some patients at these treatments were "calm, composed, and feel nothing; others cough, spit, have slight pains, feel a glow locally or all over the body, accompanied by perspiration; others are shaken and tormented by convulsions."

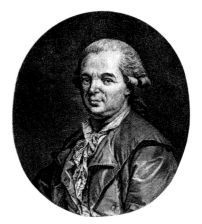

Dr. Franz Anton Mesmer (1734–1815) reintroduced to Western scientific medicine an association between trance and healing known in many cultures worldwide. Mesmer's work went against the rationalist spirit of his age, and he was condemned by the medical establishments of Vienna and then Paris. His ideas live on in Western medicine in the use of hypnosis for pain control and other healing.

Commission members witnessed "piercing cries, tears, hiccoughs, and extravagant laughter. The convulsions are preceded and followed by a state of languor and reverie, by exhaustion and drowsiness."

Critical observers discovered in Mesmer's treatments more hysteria than science and no small measure of sexual stimulation. Mesmer was denounced as a charlatan, and the king's commission agreed with this conclusion. The commissioners tested the metal rods and found no tug of magnetism. They proclaimed that the many reported cures arose from the imaginations of his patients: "Imagination without magnetism produces convulsions but magnetism without imagination produces nothing."

But one commission member—Dr. Antoine-Laurent de Jussieu, a well-known botanist—issued a minority report. Whatever the validity of Mesmer's theories and theatrical treatments, Jussieu was convinced that *something* in Mesmer's trances had effected inexplicable cures, if only by mobilizing the imagination of his patients. Benjamin Franklin, in part, seemed to agree with Jussieu. As commission chairman, he put his name to the majority report but was fascinated to think that belief might induce bodily effects. Following the royal commission's report, Mesmer's star fell into eclipse. He left us with two English words: *mesmerism*, describing his science, and *mesmerize*, meaning "to hypnotize, to enthrall." And "animal magnetism" has come to mean the kind of personal presence Mesmer himself must have possessed.

The Mysteries of Hypnosis

There was, of course, nothing revolutionary in Mesmer's healing sessions. Individual and group trance have been associated with healing across

The woman on the left is receiving Mesmeric "passes" across her body. Investigators could find no evidence of magnetism in Mesmer's "magnetic" paraphernalia.

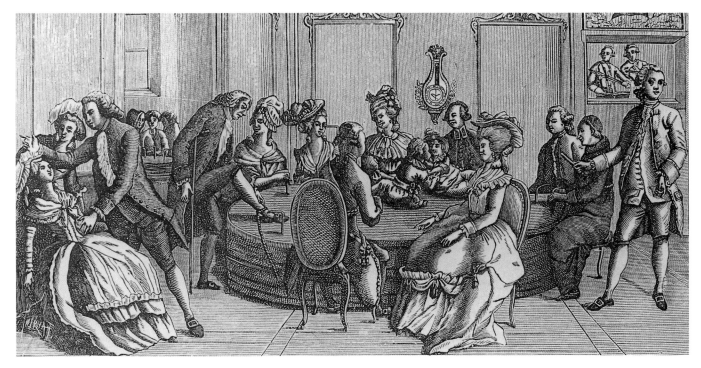

Approximately 70 percent of people are hypnotizable to one degree or another. Mind-body scientists are particularly fascinated with the approximately 4 percent of the population classified as highly hypnotizable—those who seem most able to translate mental image into bodily change. Dr. Herbert Spiegel, a psychiatrist and hypnosis specialist at Columbia University, believes these people share certain characteristics. They are generally trusting, able to suspend critical judgment, and able to get involved mentally in new events. They can concentrate, possess excellent memories, and tend to focus on the present.

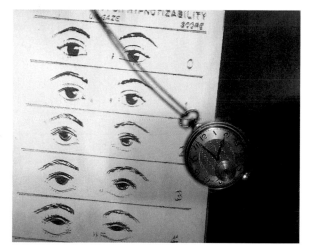

In 1968, Spiegel devised an eye-roll test for hypnotizability. First, subjects are asked to roll their eyes upward. Then, while maintaining that eye position, they are asked slowly to lower their eyelids. The more the white of the eye is visible just before the eyelids close, the more likely that the person is able to enter a trance.

In one study, psychologists S. C. Wilson and T. X. Barber surveyed twenty-seven highly hypnotizable women and concluded that they were first-rate imaginers, able to lose themselves in a world of fantasy. Most of these women would have been called daydreamers as children—they were prone to imaginative activities such as reading, make-believe play, and theatrical games. Many had shared the company of an imaginary playmate. From early childhood these women had been profoundly aware of touch, smell, taste, and other sensory experiences. Most possessed vivid memories of their lives from before the age of two, and many claimed to have had telepathic, extrasensory, or other paranormal experiences. As adults they remained prone to fantasy. The researchers believed that this ability to imagine was directly related to the women's ability to convert mental images to physical reality—a skill often referred to as *mind-body plasticity*.

How powerful are the physical changes exerted by these imaginings? The majority of women in the survey reported sensitivity to imagined heat and cold as if it were the real thing. One woman told of having to bundle up in blankets in her already warm living room while watching a portion of the movie *Doctor Zhivago* that takes place in Siberia. Another reported vomiting in a movie theater because she identified so strongly with an on-screen character who was drinking beer in a bouncing pickup truck.

Most of the women reported being able to trigger sexual orgasm with mental images, without physical stimulation. Sixty percent had experienced false pregnancies accompanied by such very real physical symptoms as breast changes, abdominal enlargement, morning sickness, and cravings for specific foods. Two of the women actually sought abortions for these pregnancies; in the others the symptoms subsided in the face of test results that the pregnancies were false.

No one knows why highly hypnotizable subjects so easily and completely lose themselves in imagination. Some studies suggest that this tendency is inborn and may be related to brain function. Whatever its cause, the tendency may not always be an advantage. Some researchers believe that such highly imaginative people are most at risk for developing multiple personality disorder under the pressure of intense childhood abuse.

many of the world's cultures. Unfortunately, the link between trance and healing has received little attention from Western scientists. In our time, as in Mesmer's, the medical establishment tends to write off trance healing as irrational superstition, which works—if it works at all—because of the patient's imagination.

The single exception is hypnosis, which may be seen as the maturation of Mesmer's ideas in Western medicine. Psychiatrists and psychotherapists use hypnosis to help patients recall experiences buried in the unconscious and to cure addictions. Some medical doctors use hypnosis to treat muscle strains, burns, asthma, and skin conditions.

Like placebo healing, hypnotic healing often involves the suggestion that physical change will take place. In hypnosis, that suggestion is often offered by a doctor or hypnotist, after putting the person in a trance state, which may heighten suggestibility. We all know the cliché: "Look *d-e-e-p* into my eyes, you are getting *v-e-r-y s-l-e-e-p-y*." Doctors also can induce hypnosis in much less dramatic ways, with a simple snap of the fingers, for example.

In fact, a person does not go to sleep at all during hypnosis, but remains awake in a state of concentrated, focused relaxation. The hypnotic state, like similar states of consciousness, is simply a special way of paying attention that is not imposed from the outside but arises from inside the mind. Some people seem more capable than others of "paying attention" in this special way, and many people can hypnotize themselves. The hypnotist—when there is one—may simply set the stage and act as guide.

One of the first medical uses of hypnosis was to provide relief from the terrible pain of surgery before the discovery of ether, chloroform, and other anesthetic drugs. In the 1860s, a British surgeon, James Esdaile, reported that he performed hundreds of successful, pain-free surgeries under so-called mesmeric anesthesia. Dr. Esdaile amputated arms and

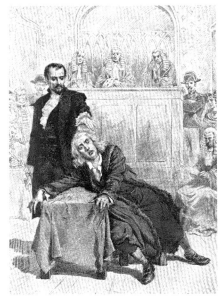

breasts and excised tumors. He sliced out cataracts, drained abscesses, and pulled teeth.

A journalist named F. W. Sims once watched Esdaile amputate the leg of a hypnotized woman in India. Sims was particularly surprised at how little the wound bled and at how still the woman lay. Esdaile sliced through the flesh and sawed the bone a little below the knee. "During the whole operation," Sims wrote, "not the least movement or change in her limbs, body, or countenance took place: she continued in the same apparently easy repose as at first, and I have no reason to believe she was not perfectly at ease."

Anesthesia and pain relief remain among the most common medical uses of hypnosis. Sometimes hypnosis is used because a patient fears or is allergic to anesthetic drugs. A 1979 review of medical literature discovered two dozen such surgeries over the previous twenty years—including an appendectomy, a Cesarean section, and several kinds of heart surgery—all performed under hypnotic trance without drugs or anesthesia. Victor Rausch, an Ontario dentist who routinely uses hypnosis in his practice, reported in the *American Journal of Clinical Hypnosis* that he had hypnotized himself for gallbladder surgery. The doctors sliced Rausch open, removed his gallbladder, then sewed him back up again. When they were done, Rausch calmly rose from the operating table and walked back to his room.

Only about 15 percent of patients are "susceptible" enough to hypnosis to undergo painful operations without anesthetic drugs. In other patients, hypnosis may allow the use of less anesthesia or postoperative pain medication. Since the side effects of pain medication can be hard to tolerate for long periods of time, patients with chronic pain may also benefit from hypnosis. It has been used to help control lower-back pain and pain from ulcers, dental extractions, and migraine headaches.

Unlike placebos, hypnosis does not seem to relieve

pain through the release of endorphins, the brain's own morphinelike drugs. Experiments have shown that hypnotic anesthesia is not reversed by naloxone, the drug that counteracts endorphin-induced pain control. Under hypnosis, the pain is not so much blocked as it is profoundly ignored. Patients are aware of the pain without experiencing it as painful.

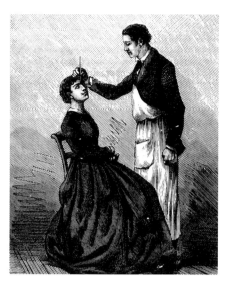

The Sensitive Skin

Modification of pain is not the only bodily change resulting from hypnotic suggestion. Hypnosis particularly affects the skin, the largest organ of the body. This shouldn't surprise us since messages from the mind seem particularly able to affect the skin. We all blush when we are embarrassed and flush red when we are angry. Under hypnosis, the effects of the mind on the skin may be more dramatic.

A case reported in the *American Journal of Clinical Hypnosis* in 1966 provides a good illustration. The "victim," in what a mystery writer might call "The Case of the Sunless Sunburn," was a young woman undergoing psychotherapy. During a session her psychotherapist hypnotized her, and then, to relax her, he innocently asked her to imagine she was on a sunny beach. Almost immediately, the woman cried out in pain, "I feel like I'm on fire," and an angry rash erupted on her face, shoulders, and upper arms. The therapist then touched the woman's skin, which felt very hot. The story later came out that the woman had previously suffered exactly such a reaction during a visit to a beach, possibly because of a drug she was taking. Her hypnotic reaction looked and felt like the real thing and lasted for eighteen hours.

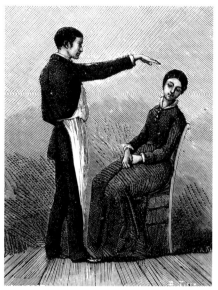

This is not a one-of-a-kind story. Other hypnotists have reported the reappearance in hypnotized patients of former burns and wounds. Sometimes new wounds are created as well, simply by the power of the mind. In one instance a hypnotized woman was "burned" on the arm by an ordinary coin after her hypnotist suggested that the coin was red hot.

Opposite page: Today doctors use hypnosis to treat several illnesses and addictions. But when it was introduced in the nineteenth century, hypnosis — or Mesmerism, as it was called — was often regarded as an entertaining parlor trick. This page: Many experts now believe that hypnosis produces a special but not uncommon state of consciousness that many people can bring on themselves. This illustration, from an earlier era, depicts one view of the stages of hypnosis and illustrates the mystery that has long surrounded the procedure.

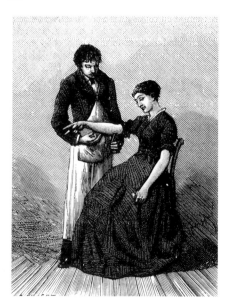

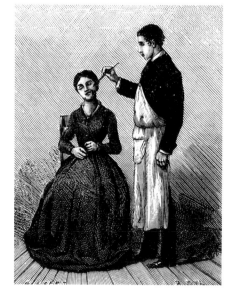

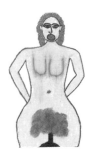

One way to test the mind's influence on healing would be to observe identical bodies inhabited by different minds. Although such research is impossible in the laboratory, a similar model already exists in persons suffering from multiple personality disorder, or MPD. This rare psychological condition begins in childhood, almost always as a reaction to extreme abuse. By adulthood, the same body may accommodate two personalities or two dozen, each with a different memory of its own history. Without therapy, the "host personality," which occupies the body most of the time, may have no knowledge that the other personalities even exist. Such disorders are called "dissociative" because the afflicted person "dissociates," or separates, from the host personality. The books *Sybil, The Three Faces of Eve*, and *The Minds of Billy Milligan* are all true stories about persons with MPD—sometimes called simply "multiples."

Therapists have learned to expect radical physical changes in a multiple when one personality disappears and another emerges. In shifting from a female personality to one that is male, for example, the voice may drop, the carriage and walk may coarsen, the gestures may become dramatically heavier and more masculine. In the same individual, one personality may require eyeglasses while the others do not, or one may be left-handed while the others are right-handed. If a multiple is also diabetic, one personality may require more insulin than another.

Some of the most dramatic differences between the personalities of a multiple involve allergies. Dr. Bennett Braun, founder of the nation's first in-patient unit for dissociative

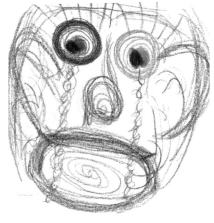

disorders, at Rush Presbyterian Hospital in Chicago, reported on a patient who was allergic to cats in one personality and not another. In another case, a boy was allergic to orange juice in all but one of his almost dozen personalities. The boy could drink orange juice and digest it in this personality, but if he switched too soon to an allergic one, he would break out in a rash, which would in turn disappear if he switched back to the nonallergic personality.

Multiples may also demonstrate the kinds of skin reactions sometimes displayed under hypnosis. Dr. Braun told of noticing red marks on the skin of a young woman during therapy. Some of the marks were triangular, others circular, and they were about the circumference of a cigarette. Over the next weeks the marks returned when, and only when, the woman assumed one particular personality. While in this personality, the woman told Braun that the marks were burns, and Braun was able to confirm that the woman had been tortured as a child by having cigarettes extinguished on her skin. The marks appeared in only one personality because that was the one "in control" of the child when she was burned.

Many therapists believe that multiples heal more quickly than other people. And some multiples seem to have one personality specifically identified as "healer." This raises the question of whether multiples hold some secret of inner healing. In fact, many of the bodily changes multiples display occur also in normal subjects under hypnosis—and even without hypnosis in some instances. We need to learn much more about multiples. The more we learn, the closer we will be to understanding how their remarkable capacities may relate to the capacities of people without dissociative disorders.

Donna Marlow, who was diagnosed as having multiple personality disorder in 1990, had, until then, been misdiagnosed as having schizophrenia. The art on these two pages were created by four different personalities. Opposite page: *Evergreen* (left) depicts rebirth and the healing process, affirming that healing is possible. *Past is Present* (middle) depicts the sudden emergence of memory, which blurs the boundaries of past and present. This page: In *Once Upon a Windy Day* (top) the creation of different personalities (called splitting) is shown as flight or escape from traumatic events. The plant "beings" in *The Guardians* (bottom) express the need for protection and also are the keepers of memories.

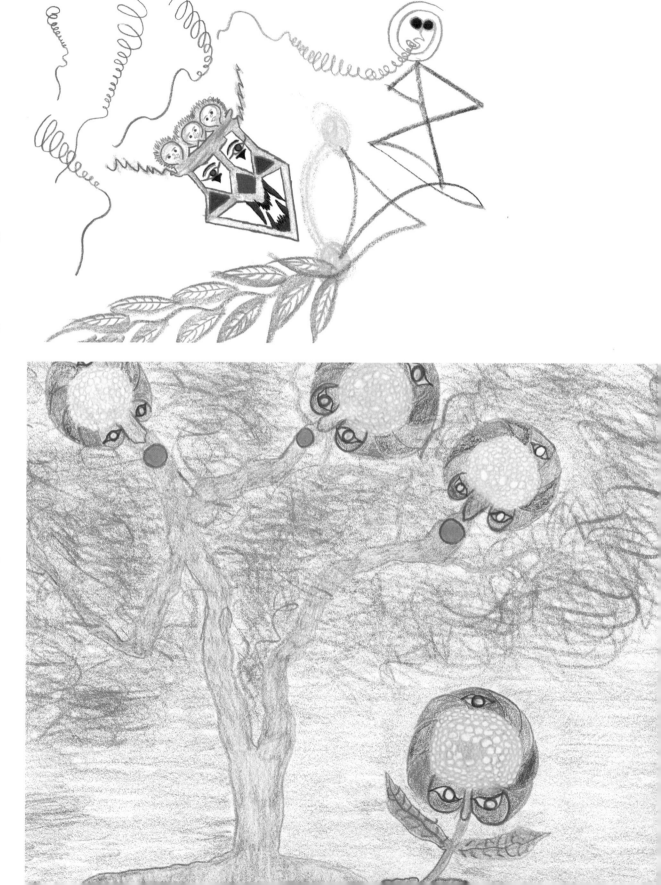

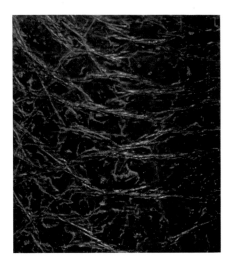

A patch of skin exhibits ichthyosiform erythroderma, commonly called "fish-skin disease," a condition that can be remarkably responsive to hypnotic suggestion, as are many skin conditions.

In another case the "burning" was accomplished with a pencil. In both experiments a blister rose in exactly the place where the object had been pressed. Such tabloid wonders suggest that some persons, under some conditions, possess a remarkable ability to transform mental images into biological fact. No one can be certain how this works, except to suggest that in a very few hypnotizable people the suggested burn is experienced as genuine and the skin reacts as it would to a genuine burn. Some researchers have suggested that not only must the subjects be hypnotizable, but they also must have experienced a real burn.

Building on the knowledge that hypnosis can sometimes create burns, some hypnotists treat genuine burns through prompt hypnotic suggestion. The idea is essentially the same, except that instead of suggesting that the patient imagine heat, the hypnotist suggests cool and healing. Dr. Dabney Ewin, a physician and hypnotist in New Orleans, has been treating burn patients in this way since the 1970s. In a case reported in 1978, a worker fell into 950-degree molten lead up to his knees. Usually such an injury would produce the extensive tissue destruction of third-degree burns, requiring skin grafts and lengthy hospitalization. But the worker was highly hypnotizable and was rushed to Dr. Ewin immediately after the injury. Instead of third-degree burns, only second-degree burns resulted. No skin grafting was required, and the man left the hospital after only three weeks.

At the burn unit of Alta Bates Hospital, in Berkeley, California, Dr. Jerold Kaplan and Dr. Lawrence Moore devised a way to test the degree to which hypnosis is responsible for helping burns. Five patients were selected who had been burned equally on both sides of their bodies, enabling the doctors to direct healing suggestions to one side but not the other. In four of the five patients, healing was more advanced in the areas to which the hypnotic suggestion was directed.

Some skin diseases also respond well to hypnotic suggestion. A famous case in the 1940s involved an unhappy English boy who suffered from ichthyosiform erythroderma, more colorfully known as "fish-skin disease." This rare, progressive disease is generally thought to be incurable. Patients suffer from dark, scaly skin, sometimes as hard as fingernails and so thick and inflexible that it cracks and bleeds. Bacteria can infect the cracks in the skin, causing a noxious odor. In this case, the fish skin covered the boy's feet, legs, and buttocks and extended up his back and down his arms to envelop his hands. The boy smelled so bad he was no longer able to attend school. Several doctors had tried and failed to relieve the boy's misery with salves. Then a physician and hypnotist, A. A. Mason, took over the case. Mason placed the boy under hypnosis. "Concentrate on your left arm," he instructed, "feel the skin becoming normal." Within five days, the horny hide on that arm—and that arm only—softened and sloughed off. During the next weeks, Mason shifted the boy's focus from one body part to the next. The scales fell off the boy's arms, from 90 percent of his back, and from 50 to 70 percent of his

Can people choose to die on one day rather than another? Folklore has long suggested that they can. Stories abound about people waiting to die until a job has been completed or a child has been married or graduated from college. And scientific studies going back fifty years confirm that the timing of death may be related to the anniversary of a significant life event.

Some of these anniversaries carry particular dread. Some research suggests, for example, that a person may become sick or die upon reaching the age at which his or her father or mother died. Researchers call these painful anniversaries "deadlines."

Other anniversaries, called "lifelines," may be anticipated with more pleasure than pain. For example, three early U.S. presidents—all signers of the Declaration of Independence—died on the Fourth of July, the anniversary of that document. John Adams and Thomas Jefferson

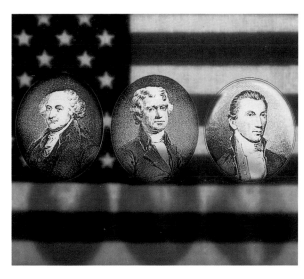

died on July 4, 1826, the fiftieth anniversary of the signing, and Jefferson is said to have inquired of his doctor, "Is it the Fourth?" shortly before he died. James Monroe had been in decline for months before his death on July 4, 1831, and it was reported at the time that he seemed to "have lingered until this time to add to the number of revolutionary patriots whose deaths have occurred on this memorable anniversary."

Researchers recently studied the deaths of elderly Chinese-American women around the time of the Harvest Moon Festival—a holiday in which older women play a central and honored role. A review of California death certificates (from 1960 to 1984) by David Phillips, a sociologist at the University of California, San Diego, found a 35.1 percent decrease in the deaths of these women in the week before the festival. Immediately after the festival, the deaths briefly climbed nearly 35 percent. There was no observed effect among old Chinese men or young Chinese women. In another study, Phillips found a similar pattern among deaths of Jewish men during the period surrounding Passover, as if these people were waiting to die until after the holiday was over. It is interesting to note that deaths from cardiovascular disease appeared to show the most fluctuations around significant occasions in both the Harvest Moon study and the Passover study.

Birthdays can also affect the timing of death—but not as strongly as holidays, perhaps because people do not think of their birthdays in as consistent a way as they do holidays. In one study, researchers examined twelve years' worth of California death certificates and found that women were about 3 percent more likely to die in the week following their birthday than in any other week of the year. Men, by contrast, were more likely to die in the few weeks before their birthday. A birthday may function as a "lifeline" for women, the researchers suggested, and as more of a "deadline" for men.

Some people may consciously will themselves to live until after a holiday or birthday—and perhaps even strike a bargain with God to go peacefully after the event is over. In others, controlling the day of death may be unconscious. In either case, such control reflects an ability to manage bodily processes that few people understand they possess.

legs and buttocks. Mason's account of the case in the *British Medical Journal* attracted so much interest that the journal had to open an additional telephone switchboard to handle the calls. Other physicians and hypnotists have since duplicated Mason's success.

Some skin conditions are caused by allergies. Many people erupt in a rash after eating certain foods or touching certain animals, plants, or chemical-laden products. Most people are allergic to poisonous plants, such as poison ivy or poison oak. We assume that something in our bodies makes us allergic to these plants—that we either react to them or we do not.

But skin allergies are not so simple, as Dr. Yujiro Ikemi and Dr. Shunji Nakagawa reported in 1962 after they tested thirteen boys known to be allergic to a Japanese plant similar to poison ivy. Five of the boys were hypnotized formally, the others simply treated with "strong suggestion." Two tests followed. First the boys' arms were rubbed with a harmless plant, which they were told was the poisonous one. Then each boy was rubbed with the poisonous plant but told it was harmless. The results suggest once more the power of the mind in altering what we assume to be a straightforward physical response. Eleven of the thirteen boys failed to react with their customary blisters and itching to the poisonous plant, but each boy developed a rash from the harmless one.

Warts may be the most common skin condition treated with hypnosis. These harmless but embarrassing skin growths are caused by a common virus. Doctors frequently burn off warts or freeze them with chemicals, but almost as frequently the warts return. Under hypnosis, however, some patients can not only cure intractable warts but clear them on one side of the body, if that's where the hypnotist directs them to concentrate. A typical cure was reported in 1973 in the *Archives of General Psychiatry*. A young girl named Holly developed her first wart soon after she had entered grammar school. For three years, doctors were unable to halt the steady advance of warts across Holly's hands and face. By the time the girl agreed to hypnosis, she was suffering from thirty-one warts and was being teased almost unbearably at school. Holly viewed the hypnosis as a game. Her hypnotist told her to concentrate on feeling the warts tingle. After the warts tingled, she was told, they

would go away. And they did begin to go away—after the very first session. After five months, only two small warts remained.

Many of us carry the virus for warts, but only a few of us break out in the disease. Why is this? What switch activates the virus in some people and not in others, and how is hypnosis able to flip off this switch? We don't know, but we do know that hypnotists and others are able to cure many cases of warts using the power of suggestion. This may account for the reported success of folk remedies for the condition.

In the 1920s, Dr. Bruno Bloch, the renowned wart doctor of Zurich, treated warts with a phony but theatrical machine, which featured flashing lights and a clamorous motor and supposedly bombarded the warts with poisonous rays. After treating his patients with the machine, Bloch would paint their warts with a harmless dye that was not to be washed off or even touched until the growths had disappeared. This treatment was successful, Bloch reported, in 31 percent of his cases.

In his book *Health and Healing*, Dr. Andrew Weil relates a story of a contemporary wart-killing machine. The patient was a man in his fifties who had suffered for years from warts over most of his body. All standard treatments had failed. Finally, the man's physician told him about a new, powerful, potentially dangerous form of x-ray treatment that might help. The patient undressed and stood in a darkened x-ray room. The x-ray machine snapped on and hummed impressively but in fact did not emit a single ray. The next day all of the warts simply melted away. "The doctor was impressed," Weil wrote, "but it never occurred to him to try to find out what went on in the patient's mind-body or to consider the implications of what he had seen."

Cancer physician and writer Lewis Thomas proposed a national effort to study the mental cure of warts. "Just think of what we would know, if we had anything like a clear understanding of what goes on when a wart is hypnotized away," Thomas said. He spoke of an inner "controller . . . a kind of superintelligence that exists in each of us." To discover this healing superintelligence "would be worth a War on Warts, a Conquest of Warts, a National Institute of Warts and All."

How Hypnosis May Affect the Body

We do have some hints about how hypnotic suggestion may result in physical effects. One way hypnosis seems to work is by controlling blood flow, which could, for example, rush healing nutrients to burned tissue or choke off the nutrition to warts. Hypnosis can control blood flow so well it is often used to stop the bleeding from surgery or dental work.

Hypnosis may also effect changes by altering the body's immune function, which is responsible for protecting against viral diseases such as warts, as well as every other disease, from colds to cancer. By altering immune function, hypnosis may also alter allergic reactions, which are overreactions of the immune system to a perceived threat.

That hypnosis can alter immune function has been demonstrated simply by hypnotizing subjects and giving them a tuberculin skin test. Most of us have received this test, in which a tiny sample of inactivated tuberculosis bacteria is injected beneath the skin. A positive tuberculin test—a raised, red weal on the skin—is an immune response demonstrating previous exposure to the bacteria. Under hypnosis, however, this biological response can be substantially modified. Under hypnotic suggestion not to react, some previously positive subjects will produce a much reduced response to the tuberculin. Other subjects, when told they will react, produce a red weal when given an injection of water. Most incredible, both "false" reactions have been produced in the same person at the same time. Altering blood flow and immune function are only two of many ways hypnosis may effect bodily change. Other systems may be involved. We simply have not mapped the intricacies of the mind-body connection.

But what of the hypnotic state? What is it about trance that prompts bodily reactions? It is tempting to think of hypnosis as a kind of super-placebo, since both placebos and hypnosis involve suggestion. But studies have found no relationship between a person's susceptibility to placebos and his or her susceptibility to hypnosis. True hynotizability is a life-long characteristic that seems to involve both an ability to concentrate and a vivid, engaging imagination. Such persons are able to imagine so strongly that they have access to their minds in profoundly special ways. How rare is this capacity? Are there degrees of hypnotizability? How is being hypnotized similar to other states of consciousness, such as profound relaxation, religious trance, or the kind of mass trance of healing ceremonies in other cultures? Is there a way to induce these states of consciousness to affect our own health? We will come back to these questions in later chapters. For now, hypnosis cures are one more piece of evidence that at the heart of healing lie mysteries we have yet to comprehend.

Western medicine has mostly ignored the power of the mind in health and disease. One exception is hypnosis, which has had a role in Western medicine since the late nineteenth century. Here, a group of French doctors in the 1890s watch a colleague put a patient into a hypnotic trance.

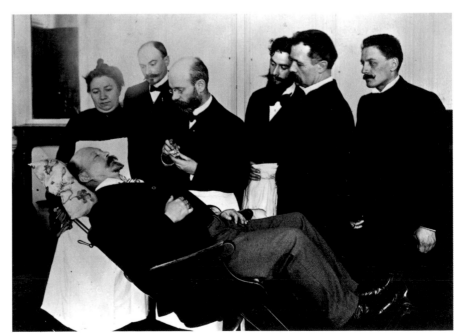

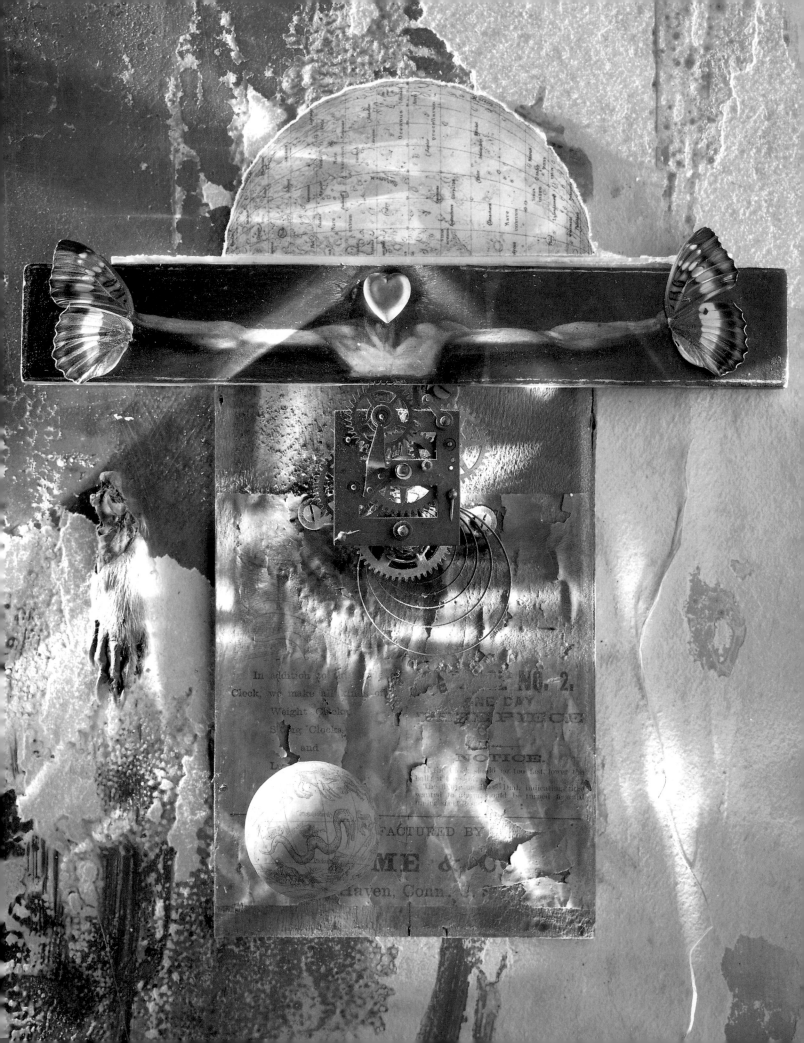

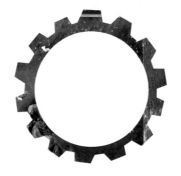

CHAPTER TWO

HEALING AND CULTURE

FROM SHAMAN TO SHINY MEDICAL MACHINE

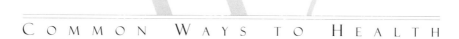

COMMON WAYS TO HEALTH

WHAT IS HEALTH?

What makes us sick? Who or what can make us well? The answers to such questions vary radically depending on when and where you ask them.

In the highlands of south-central Africa, a woman with a sore shoulder seeks out a native healer. The healer listens to the woman's complaint. Then, slipping into a trance, he becomes the spirit of the woman's long-dead grandmother and in a high, quavering voice diagnoses his patient's condition. The sore shoulder is a result of jealousy, the "grandmother" expounds through the healer. In the midst of the most serious drought in living memory, as crops shrivel in the fields, the woman has continued to live well on grain she set aside in previous years. Her neighbors are resentful, and one of them has put a hex on her, filling her body with evil spirits.

Dramatically, the healer sniffs the woman up and down until he locates the offending spirits. Then, in a gesture widespread among spirit healers worldwide, he makes a sucking noise as if he is inhaling the spirits into his own body. Finally, he turns away abruptly, as he half-vomits, half-sneezes the evil essence out on the ground.

"Health depends on a state of equilibrium among the various factors that govern the operation of the body and the mind; the equilibrium in turn is reached only when man lives in harmony with his external environment." —HIPPOCRATES (460?-377? B.C.)

How silly, some people might think, how irrational. How could evil spirits create a physical symptom such as a sore shoulder? How can trance and sniffing be used to diagnose disease?

In a Western hospital a sore shoulder is often x-rayed and is sometimes put through a computerized scan. Depending on the results, the patient is diagnosed as having a muscle pull, tendonitis, arthritis, or a compressed nerve. A physician might prescribe pain medication or inject cortisone into the joint to fight inflammation. If that didn't work, the patient might end up in surgery.

Those who have grown up with Western medicine tend to make assumptions about Western versus non-Western approaches to disease and treatment. They judge one to be modern and the other primitive; one scientific and the other based on crass superstition. But, as the previous chapter pointed out, patients being treated by practitioners of either approach get better for reasons that have little to do with the objective cause of the discomfort.

Try to picture yourself in a world where spirits are ever-present and ever-powerful. The idea that a resentful neighbor put a hex on you makes perfect sense. You have heard from childhood how spite and jealousy can lead to evil. The healer's reputation, his ability to become the spirit of your grandmother, the drama of the sucking ceremony—how could they fail to move you? No less moving for a Western patient are the assumptions and rituals surrounding healing in a Western setting. Everything about our culture teaches us to believe in the supremacy of technology and the Western scientific approach. In our culture, physical ailments are understood to have physical causes. The hum of the x-ray machine, the cool sterility of the examination room, the doctor's stethoscope and white coat all say "healing" to us.

If pills or injections kill the pain, it may be in part because we expect them to, in the same way that the healer's incantations may help relieve the African woman's discomfort. In both cases, much of the relief hinges on beliefs or on mechanisms of healing we do not understand. And because these beliefs lie at the heart of a culture, it is difficult for those of us in one culture to judge the approach to healing of another.

Western scientific medicine is eminently successful at treating some kinds of diseases and has much to teach the world. At the same time, some of us in the West are beginning to understand how much other cultures have to teach us. Especially revealing are the similarities in approaches to healing across cultures, for here resides our collective wisdom on health and healing. Such similarities include an association between health and spirit, belief, trance, altered states, and the concept of balance.

Spirit, Trance, and Health

There has never been a culture without a concept of health and healing. We all get sick, suffer, and seek relief. Health is basic, central to the human enterprise, inevitably linked to such other basic concepts as family, community, and religious or spiritual life. In our own language, the very word *health* is derived from the same ancient root as *whole*, *wholesome*, *hallowed*, and *holy*.

The question "Why is there illness?" is a religious or philosophical question, another way of asking "Why is there evil in the world?" This question, in turn, is linked to other philosophical puzzles, such as the purpose of life and the meaning of death.

Many people throughout the centuries have thought of health as a gift of the gods and disease as divine punishment. The ancient Egyptians, Chinese, Greeks, and people of India all worshiped constellations of gods who were believed to cause disease or intercede for those seeking cures. Similarly, Christians in medieval Europe thought disease was a punishment of God for human sin—an idea that continues to this day among some Christians.

So wedded is healing to spiritual life that the first professional health-care advisers were doctor-priests. These healers interceded with the deities or interpreted divine will as expressed in dreams and visions. Sometimes they counseled patients on physical, family, and social problems or prescribed herbal cures. And because one role of religion was—and still is—the preservation of culture and community, advice on health matters often dealt with such practical concerns as getting along with family and meeting the expectations of neighbors.

In many of the world's oldest healing traditions, spirit and health are linked in the person of a *shaman*, a magical healer of the sort who "sucked" the evil spirits from the woman with the sore shoulder. Tribal people and their descendants worldwide seek shamanistic intervention with the spirit world as a solution to all kinds of problems. In many places this tradition still thrives alongside a Western medical system. People may seek healing in both systems, or seek healing in a second system only after treatment in the first system brings no relief. Shamanistic healers are often called "witch doctors" or "medicine men," but this is a misnomer. Although some shamans are herbal healers or know how to treat traumatic injury, the shaman's realm more characteristically is the realm of the spirit and the imagination.

As anthropologist Weston La Barre has observed, the shaman is the world's oldest professional and is both a performer and a priest: "The shaman was the original artist, dancer, musician, singer, dramatist, intellectual, poet, bard, ambassador, advisor to chiefs and king, entertainer, actor and clown, curer, stage magician, juggler, jongleur, folksinger, weatherman, culture hero, and trickster-transformer."

Physician Andrew Weil, who has studied contemporary shamanism in South America, calls the shaman the "doctor of bodies, souls and situations." The shaman, Weil says, "has learned to be a personal mediator between the everyday world and the 'other world,' leaving his body to commune with spirits and learn the specific cause of illness, the whereabouts of missing objects, the reasons for failures of crops."

In the shaman's world, every disease has a cause, although most Western doctors would not recognize the cause as such. Demons and witches are thought to cause disease, as are opposing malevolent shamans. A soul can be tempted from a body through sorcery, leaving it open to illness. Objects of evil power—pebbles, crystals, even small animals—can be magically transplanted into the body, causing misery. Disease can also occur after the victim has broken some taboo.

One of the most skilled shamans Dr. Weil visited, a man named Luis, attracted patients from miles around to a remote village in southwestern Colombia. Patients journeyed for several days to reach Luis—by bus, river

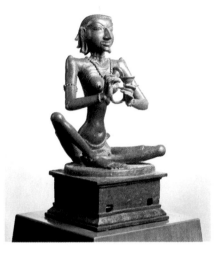

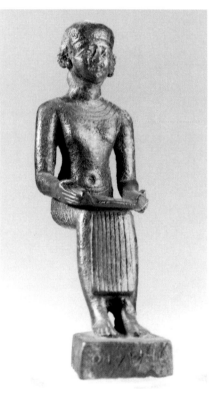

Health and disease have been associated with spirit and religion throughout the histories of most human cultures. Top: This twelfth-century copper figure shows a devotee of Kali, an Indian goddess associated with disease, death, and destruction. Bottom: A statue, almost five thousand years old, of Imhotep, Egyptian scribe, physician, poet, and architect, who was worshiped as a healing divinity.

OF HEALING

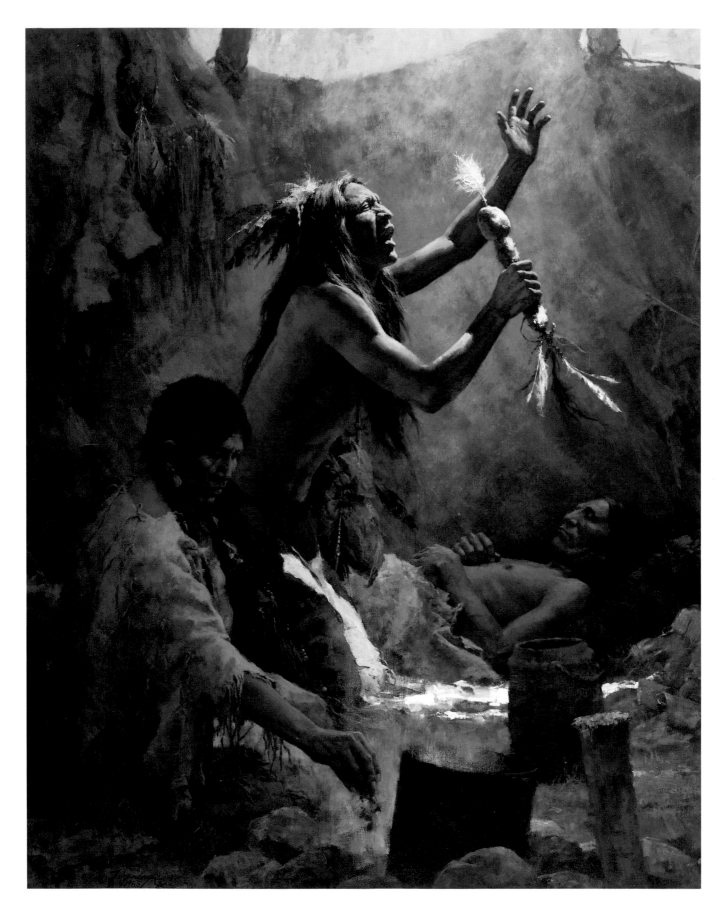

steamer, and finally on foot. Once a week, when his patients assembled, Luis would brew a hallucinogenic drink called *yagé* from the plants in the jungle. During a long night of chanting, dancing, and praying, Luis would imbibe great drafts of *yagé* and give it to his patients—some with high fevers, convulsions, infections, and paralysis. In the resulting visions, Luis would "see" the causes and cures of his patients' diseases, and in the morning he would prescribe cures for each of them—sometimes herbal remedies, sometimes commercial drugs. Interviews with Luis's patients convinced Dr. Weil that many felt they had been cured.

Luis's healing techniques were similar to those used in many cultures. The use of medicines, whether herbs or chemical drugs, is a widespread practice, and the long journey to reach Luis must have raised a patient's investment in cure, in the same way a trip to Lourdes might, or even a journey to reach the best medical specialists in America. Similarly, the elaborate ritual—the firelight, the dancing, the chanting—all conveyed Luis's healing power to his patients.

Weil believed that the *yagé* probably contributed to Luis's healing powers, because the drug caused nausea and extreme diarrhea, which might have cleansed his patients' systems of intestinal parasites, a common cause of tropical illness. But just as important, Weil believed, were the drug's hallucinogenic properties, which might have heightened the effect of the firelight, the chanting, and the dance and sensitized the patients to the suggestion of healing, almost as if they'd been hypnotized. Trance and other altered states of consciousness are central to shamanistic healing. Altered states can also be induced through dance, drumming, chanting, singing, meditation, and prayer.

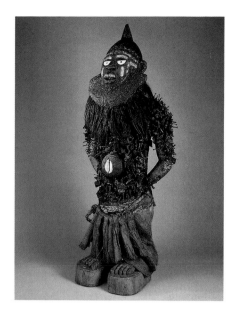

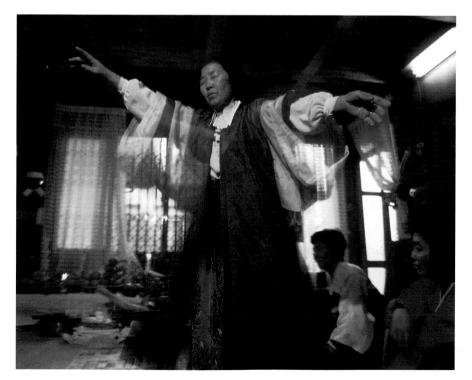

In much of the world, healing is linked to magic and the spirit realm. This page: A Bakongo nail fetish (above) is used in regions of central Africa for protection against evil spirits. A Korean shaman, a *mudang* (left), performs a ceremony, a *kut*, calling on the spirits to heal a disorder in a private home. Opposite page: The Cheyenne medicine man was a central figure in his tribe—a healer of mind, body, and spirit. Here, he performs a healing chant, while his assistant drops sweetgrass and herbs into the fire to create a purifying smoke. Although anthropologists most often apply the term *shaman* to native healers from Asia and the Americas, similar healers are found in cultures worldwide.

THE CHINESE ENERGY OF HEALTH

手厥陰心包經之圖左右二十八穴 凡九穴

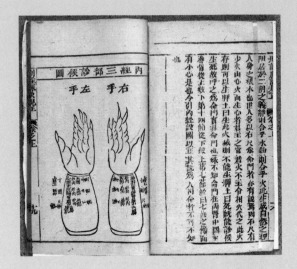

Each morning before daybreak in the major cities of China, people fill the parks and squares to practice ancient, graceful exercises known as *tai chi*. The exercises are both martial art and meditation in motion. Their purpose is to promote the flow of the body's *chi*, a vital energy said to be present throughout nature, and particularly in the early hours of daylight. *Tai chi* links the body to nature and promotes both health and spirit, which the Chinese understand to be inseparable.

A link between health and the flow of energy is found in many of the world's cultures. But perhaps no people have developed the concept as thoroughly as the Chinese, who place it at the very center of an ancient and elaborate medical system. Chinese medicine is rooted in the philosophy of its parent culture, which honors above all a state of balance, a profound, timeless stasis. Where Western medicine is concerned with identifying and conquering specific causes of disease, in Chinese medicine health is seen not as an absence of sickness but as a way of life.

It is difficult for Westerners to think about *chi*, since we have no comparable concept. Westerners talk about "vital energy," but *chi* is something more. *Chi* is movement, not the cause of movement. It is the source of growth and the process of growing. *Chi* can be seen in the flow of rivers, the accumulation of mountains, the growth of babies and children.

The idea of *chi* is closely linked to another idea in Chinese medicine, that a dynamic oneness is created by two opposite and complementary qualities called *yin* and *yang*. Like *chi*, *yin* and *yang* are everywhere in the universe. *Yin* is feminine, dark, negative, small, a characteristic of night, earth, water, and metal. *Yang* is masculine, light, positive, big, characterizing heaven, wood, and fire. Every facet of creation is a mixture of these qualities

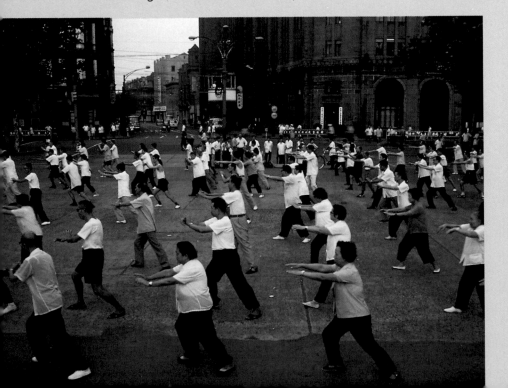

Chinese medicine is a fully developed medical science far more ancient than Western medicine. This page: A pulse chart (above) from a 1693 edition of *Secrets of the Pulse*. Residents of Shanghai (left) perform early-morning *tai chi*, which is part exercise, part meditation. Opposite page: A diagram of acupuncture points for treating the diseases of various organs dates from the Ming Dynasty (1368–1644). Acupuncture has been in continual use for thousands of years. So important is pulse taking in Chinese medicine that instead of saying "I'm going to the doctor," a patient may explain, "I am going to have my pulse felt."

flowing constantly into one another, as the dark *yin* of night flows into the light *yang* of day.

When *yin* and *yang* are in balance within a person, *chi* flows smoothly through bodily organs. When they are out of balance, the flow of *chi* is blocked. Much of Chinese medicine is based on analyzing and maximizing the flow of *chi* to the bodily organs. This flow is measured in a patient's pulses, a key diagnostic art in Chinese medicine. Some Chinese healers guide the flow of *chi* through massage or simply by fluttering their hands above a patient. Others add to or manipulate *chi* through herbal remedies or acupuncture, during which needles are inserted along energy pathways that Chinese healers call meridians. Like *chi* itself, these pathways have no counterparts in Western medicine. Meridians are neither organs nor nerves and do not survive the body's death. They are functions of energy. When *chi* leaves the body, the meridians simply disappear.

Although some of the terminology of Chinese medicine may seem similar to that of the Western system, the concepts are completely different. The stomach meridian, for example, is not located in the center of the abdomen but stretches from alongside the nose to the second toe of the left foot. Acupuncture needles are inserted along the stomach meridian not only to treat digestive disorders but to relieve headaches, mouth sores, eye problems, breast problems, and a host of other ailments.

Similarly, although Chinese doctors are able to cure many of the same medical conditions as Western doctors, these conditions are understood to arise from dramatically different causes. Chinese diagnoses often focus on the excess or deficiency of such qualities as dampness, heat, or wind and describe the overall health-illness status of the patient rather than a specific condition. A Chinese doctor might describe the Western condition peptic ulcer disease as everything from "Damp heat affecting the spleen" to "Deficient *yin* affecting

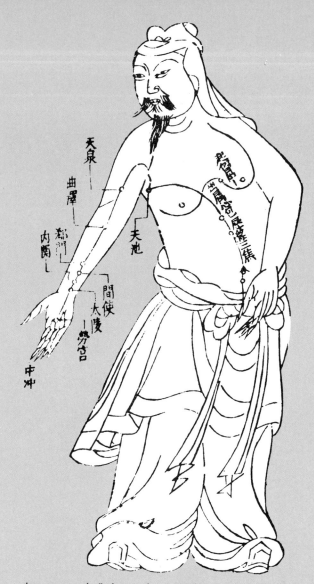

the stomach," depending on the patient's exact physical and psychological state.

Although Western medicine has made inroads in China, the native medical system is thriving. Many Chinese use both medical systems, patronizing Western doctors and hospitals for trauma care and the treatment of acute diseases, while seeking out Chinese doctors for long-term, chronic conditions. At the same time, many non-Chinese patients are now turning to Chinese medicine: visiting acupuncturists, pursuing the mindful movement exercises of *tai chi*. What seems to attract Westerners to Chinese medicine are not so much the specifics of treatment — although many have found them helpful — as the idea of an ancient medical system focusing not on the mechanical curing of diseases but on health as balance and the integration of healing into everyday life.

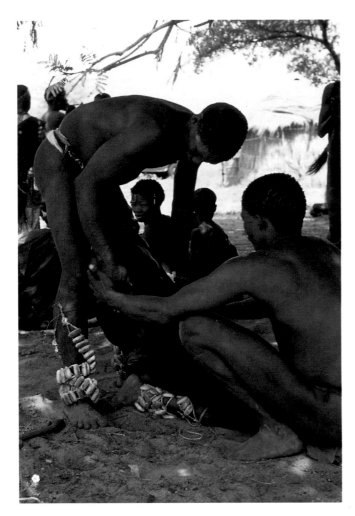

The !Kung people, a hunter-gatherer group in Africa's Kalahari Desert, also associate healing with trance. The !Kung dance, drum, and chant their way to health through a transformational healing process known as *kia*. These activities arouse in their participants a mind-body energy known as *n/um*, sometimes described as a "boiling." During *kia*, !Kung healers ceremonially put *n/um* into people to "pull out" their sickness. Some healers walk on fire (or even stick their heads directly in the flame). Some describe seeing into the bodies of their patients or "traveling to God's home."

In more familiar traditions, a Catholic priest chanting the Mass, a gospel choir shouting the Lord's praise, a Zen Buddhist deep in meditation, and a Christian penitent lost in intensive prayer may all experience a special level of consciousness that aids in healing. People who feel renewed after such religious practices may assume the renewal to be spiritual and psychological, but it may be physical as well.

A Question of Balance

Many Westerners are uncomfortable making a literal connection between spirit and healing. Over the last century we have largely turned healing over to science, with its emphasis on physical causes and physical cures of disease. We have compartmentalized our culture, assigning spirit and religion to one room and health and healing to another. This was not always so. In ancient Greece, at the dawn of the Western tradition of healing, health and disease were thought to be mediated by the gods. Those suffering from disease sought guidance in a common altered state of consciousness—their own dreams. Like visitors to Lourdes or to the shaman Luis, sick people in ancient Greece made a journey—in their case to a temple dedicated to Asclepios, the god of medicine. Once at the temple, the visitor would undergo an intricate ritual of purifying baths, sacrifices, and fasting. Then they would bed down near a statue of the god, sometimes on the skin of a ritually sacrificed animal. The priests at the temple believed that Asclepios visited the patient in a dream and offered advice, which the priests would interpret to the patient in the morning.

Such practices were standard at the time of

Healing is linked to both spiritual observance and altered mental states in many of the world's cultures. One reason people sometimes feel better after a burst of emotion may be due to chemical changes in the brain and body. Above: A !Kung man in a healing trance is held by two other !Kung men. Below: Worshipers at the Church of the Lord Jesus in Jolo, West Virginia.

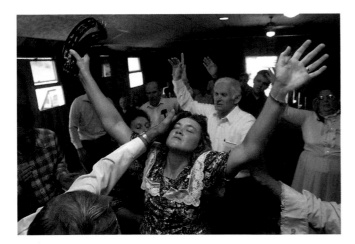

Hippocrates, a physician and teacher of medicine on the Greek island of Kos. Although there were other prominent Greek physicians at the time, Hippocrates is considered the father of Western healing and the first advocate for the rational study of disease. Hippocrates and his followers divorced medicine from magic and laid the groundwork for science. They maintained that diseases sprang from natural rather than supernatural causes and that these causes could be rationally deduced.

By Hippocrates's time, the Greeks had developed a sophisticated theory of human physiology. The body, they believed, was composed of four humors, or fluids: blood, yellow bile, black bile, and phlegm. The four humors, in turn, were manifestations of the four basic elements of the universe: water, air, fire, and spirit. Each humor carried different characteristics, and the balance of the humors within the body was thought to determine not only health and disease but also disposition. A person with excess bile, for example, was thought to have more "hot" personality characteristics and to be prone to "hot" diseases such as bacterial infection. A person with excess phlegm was thought to be "cool" and subject to "cool" diseases such as the viral congestion common in the winter that we call "colds." To this day, we also speak of a calm, sluggish person as "phlegmatic." Here then, at the very inception of Western medicine, is the first formal theory linking personality to health.

Hippocrates not only rejected magical in favor of natural causes of disease, he endorsed nature's ability to heal illnesses and restore health. "Nature heals disease," Hippocrates wrote in one early endorsement of an inner healing system. "Inherent mechanisms act automatically . . . much as the reflexes we use in winking the eyelids and moving the tongue, for nature is active without training and without schooling in the essentials." This faith would be distilled into one of the guiding precepts for early healing: *vis medicatrix naturae*, "the healing power of nature."

According to Hippocrates and other Greek physicians, a kind of life force, called *pneuma*, flowed through each individual. Hippocrates urged physicians to study not the disease but the whole patient, including the environment, emotions, and spiritual life. "Observe the nature of each country," he wrote, "the diet, customs, the age of the patient, speech, manners, fashion, even his silence, his thoughts, if he sleeps or is suffering from lack of sleep, the content and origin of his dreams. . . . One has to study all these signs and to analyze what they portend."

Halfway around the world, health practitioners in China and India had already rejected magical explanations in favor of more natural causes of health and disease. And like physicians in Greece, doctors in both China and India had come to see health as a balance of natural forces within the body. They also believed in a life force, called *prana* by the Indians and *chi* by the Chinese, which they thought needed to flow through each organ, in just the right amount, for it to function properly. Imbalances could lead to disease. One seventh-century Chinese text discusses 1,720 such diseases.

" Inherent mechanisms act automatically . . . much as the reflexes we use in winking the eyelids and moving the tongue, for nature is active without training and without schooling in the essentials."

—HIPPOCRATES

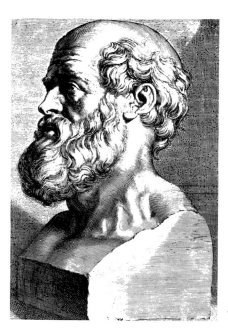

By the second century, a person dominated by one of the four humors was thought to exhibit a corresponding personality. These medieval illustrations represent men revealing the personalities associated with the four humors: sanguine, phlegmatic, melancholic, and choleric. Today, we might call them passionate, calm, sad, and bad-tempered.

That such similar systems of health evolved apparently independently suggests the power of their core concepts. The link between health and personality, the notion of health as balance, faith in the healing power of nature: the majority of the world's cultures still accept these concepts. But although the Indian and Chinese systems of health survived twenty-five centuries virtually intact, the Greek system was overwhelmed by the Western scientific revolution that began in the seventeenth century. And although hospitals specializing in Chinese or Indian medicine exist alongside Western hospitals in many Chinese and Indian cities today, there is no Hippocratic Medical Center in Paris, London, or New York.

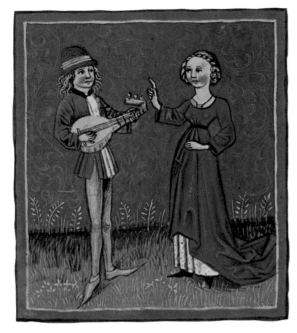

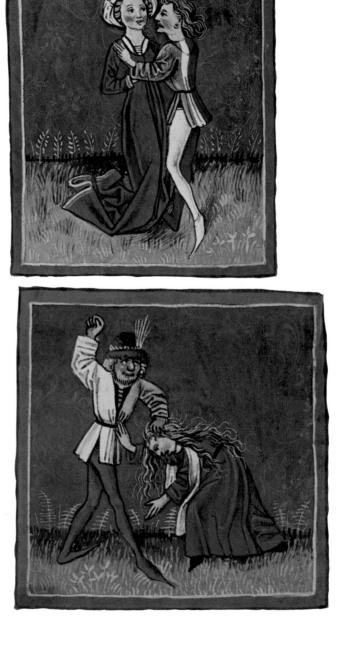

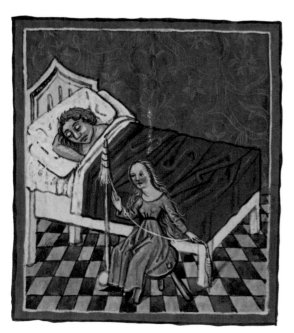

WESTERN MEDICINE AND THE MAGNIFICENT MACHINE

Hippocratic medicine survived for many centuries, largely through the agency of a second-century Greek physician named Galen, who traveled and worked in Rome and spread Hippocrates's beliefs throughout the Roman empire. Galen codified Hippocrates's teachings, expounding and expanding the humoral concept of health and disease. As a physician to the Roman gladiators, he examined wounds and created intricate anatomical drawings. He preached on the relationship between emotions and bodily ills and once estimated that 60 percent of his patients suffered from symptoms derived from emotional causes. Galen encouraged gentle therapies, such as diet, rest, and exercise, and detailed in his voluminous writings herbal treatments that are still in use today. By the Middle Ages, the teachings of Hippocrates—from Galen and enriched by Arab, Persian, and Jewish traditions of healing—were the standard medical curriculum at European universities. From the Renaissance, in the mid-sixteenth century, however, to the Age of Reason, two centuries later, one after another of the old teachings fell before an entirely new system of knowledge that became known as science.

In a public lecture in 1616, Englishman William Harvey developed the modern understanding of blood circulation, overturning the Greek notion of humors. A few years later, an Italian named Santorio Santorio used a thermometer—a brand-new invention of a countryman, Galileo—to show that bilious, or "hot,"

persons were in fact no hotter than those described as phlegmatic or "cold." If Hippocrates had established a rational basis for medicine, science now sought a more rigorous definition of "rational." No more were the human senses to be trusted. To be accepted as "true," medical facts had to be measurable and proved through an elaborate and strict system of observational rules. There was little room in this new system for collected cultural wisdom regarding health. Unprovable was the idea of health as inner balance. Unprovable was the concept that personality and spirit might affect health and disease. Immaterial to the new science was the notion of health as a reflection of culture, deeply linked to such matters as one's relationship to God (or the gods), how well one got along with family, met the expectations of neighbors, or protected the community.

Gradually, a new model of the body emerged, appropriate to the rationalistic spirit of the age. According to this model, the body is a kind of magnificent machine, the sum total of its physical parts, which work together like the finest engine. Food is understood to be fuel, which is broken down chemically and mixed with oxygen from the lungs to power cells. This fuel is circulated by the blood. Other body systems cool the machine, eliminate its waste, and move it from one place on the planet to another. The model is weighty with implications. If the body is a machine, then its mechanisms can be disassembled and analyzed to the smallest part.

Second-century Greek physician Galen was the most influential theorist of Western medicine through much of the Middle Ages. This woodcut portrait is from a text published in Venice in about 1500.

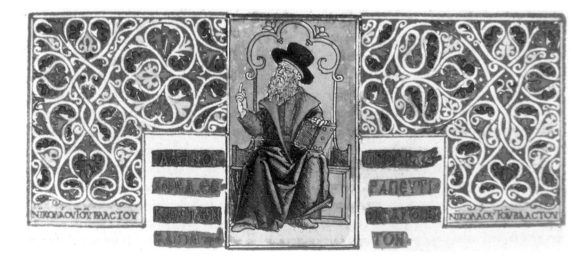

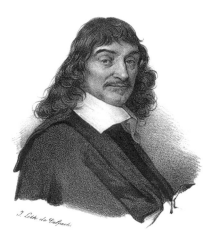

Further, a machinelike body would ultimately be understandable. And if it were understandable, it would also be predictable, independent of that most unpredictable of entities, the human mind.

The new model was particularly advanced by the work of two men, neither of whom was a doctor. The first was René Descartes, an influential seventeenth-century French philosopher. By Descartes's time the new science was locked in ongoing conflict with the all-important Roman Catholic Church. One prominent battlefield was the human body, which the church considered the reflection of God and off-limits to dissection and other scientific probing. Descartes solved this problem philosophically by asserting that the mind and body were irrevocably separate. He thus divided the human being into two parts, one part for spirit and the church and the other for worldly science. Descartes defined the mind as the holy seat of human existence. The body, by contrast, was a purely physical quantity, which would continue to function in exactly the same way "were there no mind in it at all." The human body, then,

Above: French philospher René Descartes (1596–1650) helped lay the groundwork for the Western mechanistic model of the body as machine. Clockwise from

right: Illustrations from his book *Traité de l'homme* (*Treatise on Man*): Descartes's conception of human vision, the pineal gland, and a diagram of his theory of nervous action.

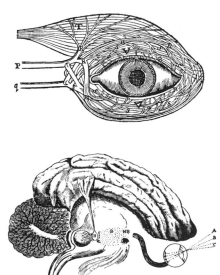

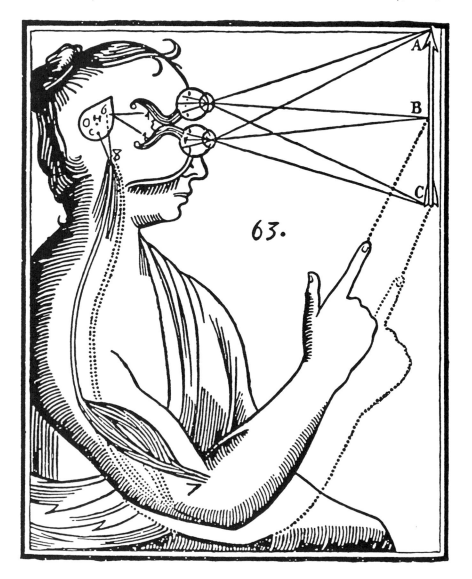

was part of nature, but the human mind became something else: an observer, an experimenter, free to manipulate and control nature.

Descartes's ideas resonated well with those of Isaac Newton. Newton, the preeminent mathematician and physicist of the mid-seventeenth centry, formulated laws of gravitation and motion that would forever change how humans thought of the world. He proposed that the universe was governed by physical laws and reduced to mechanical principles. This led to a startling new conception of the universe as a great clock, ticking away for eternity.

The themes have been repeated again and again— the body is a machine, the universe is a machine, and each is ultimately understandable by an independent mind through the study of constituent parts—in support of the scientific approach known as *reductionism*. Reductionist techniques supported the explosion of scientific inquiry beginning in the Age of Reason. Eventually, they would lead to the Industrial Revolution, the splitting of the atom, and the invention of the digital computer.

New Model, New Medicine

As in science, the advances in medicine have been remarkable. We can now cure many infectious diseases and reassemble bodies broken as a result of accidents and other traumas. Through our understanding of physiology, we have learned to support an ailing body with feeding tubes, intravenous drugs and fluids, even mechanical breathing until either that body dies or nature somehow knits it back to health.

Medicine has unlocked the structure of the cell, the chromosome, and the gene. It has engineered (and our doctors regularly transplant) some two hundred artificial body parts—everything from hip joints to heart valves—a complete set of which is now estimated to be worth $25 million. Using diagnostic tools and tests, we can now peer into the vessels of the heart, the control rooms of the cells, and the secret passages of the brain.

These medical wonders do not occur without costs, however. There are financial costs, of course—almost $2 billion a day in 1991 in the United States alone— but there are psychological and spiritual costs as well.

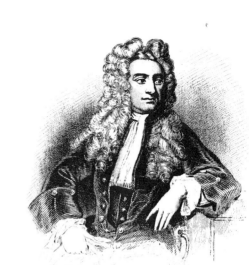

Right: Isaac Newton (1642–1727) postulated a machinelike universe that worked like a great clock. He was a philosopher as well as a mathematician and physicist, and his curiosity stretched into many areas. Below: His drawing depicting the parts of a telescope.

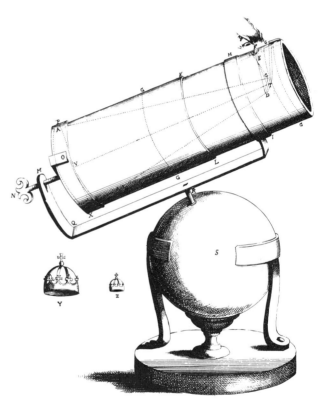

The use of medicines in healing is central in cultures worldwide. Tens of thousands of years ago, certain plants gained reputations as medicines, perhaps because they were high in vitamins or minerals or because they created chemical changes in the human body. Other plants also have acquired spiritual or symbolic healing properties.

Until the nineteenth century most Western medicines were given in the form of crude preparations of plant leaves, roots, or flowers. Plants and plant parts were often mixed together and were frequently prepared as teas. Such preparations, often given to maintain or restore bodily balance, remain the dominant form of medicine in the world today. Indian and Chinese medicine depend extensively on herbal preparations. Throughout Africa and much of the Americas and Asia plants gathered in the wild form the backbone of native healing.

Today, approximately 75 percent of Western drugs come from plants. But rather than being given whole, plants are now sought for their active ingredients. Commercial, refined drugs have their advantages. Popping pills is more convenient than chewing herbs. Refined compounds can also be measured and prescribed more precisely. But refined drugs are not always better than the preparations of the crude plants from which they come. In some cases the pharmacological effect of a plant is not due to a single active compound but to a complex mixture of interacting substances. The process of isolating and concentrating the active ingredient can make the drug more toxic than the plant. In general, commercial drugs work more quickly and affect the body more intensely than their whole-plant equivalents, but herbal medicines often are more subtle in their action, may work more slowly, and can be used longer with fewer side effects.

The Western medicines digoxin and digitoxin are derived from plants of the genus *Digitalis*, including the foxglove plant. As either plant or refined medicine, *Digitalis* compounds slow and strengthen the heart, circulating the blood and reducing swelling in the feet and ankles. As far back as A.D. 1000, female herbalists in the British Isles brewed a tea containing foxglove leaves to reduce swelling of the feet in pregnant women. Today, digoxin and digitoxin are among the most important, powerful, and widely used drugs for treating heart problems. They are potentially so toxic, however, that patients are taught how to count their heart rate before taking them. An overdose of either drug can lead to a fatally irregular heartbeat.

Many modern drugs come from herbs. Native Americans brewed tea from the bark of willows for its analgesic and fever-reducing properties. Pharmaceutical chemists later isolated salicylic acid, the active compound in willow, and incorporated it into a new drug that they called aspirin (left). While aspirin is more powerful and faster in relieving pain than willow bark tea, it is also more irritating to the stomach. Dried preparations of the foxglove plant used to be given to people with heart disease to slow and steady their heartbeats. In the twentieth century, chemists purified some active ingredients of the plant to create the common heart drugs digitalis and digoxin (right).

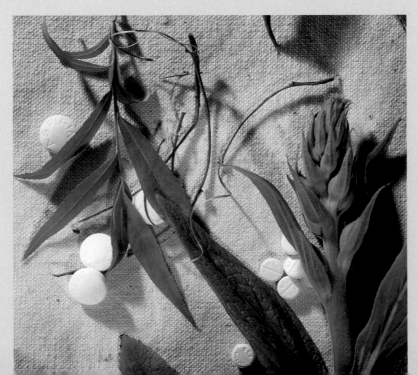

This danger did not exist before the twentieth century. Before then, *Digitalis* was given as crushed foxglove leaves in gelatin capsules, and the leaves contained an additional compound that would produce nausea and vomiting long before irregular heartbeats could begin. If a patient complained of such symptoms, a physician would simply reduce the dose to a safe level. In digoxin and digitoxin, this "safety compound" is carefully removed.

The shift from the use of herbal preparations to refined drugs reflects broader themes in Western medicine: a movement from natural to chemical treatments, the reductionist urge to seek single mechanical cures for single-cause diseases. Western medicine has come to think of medicines not as gentle tonics or correctives for the maintenance of internal balance but as magic bullets targeted at specific bodily functions or diseases.

Chemists will continue to refine drugs from natural sources and to manipulate them into entirely new pharmacoactive compounds. Some will undoubtedly be valuable drugs on which a portion of our healing science will depend. Others may present dangers as grave as the diseases they were developed to cure.

Lately, there has been a revival of interest in herbal medicine. In a rapidly shrinking world, Westerners are being exposed to Asian and other medical practices that rely on whole-plant medicines. At the same time, many people in our own culture long for a more natural, gentle, Earth-centered approach to healing.

More than two hundred years ago, the French writer Voltaire held forth caustically on the use of drugs in medicine: "Physicians pour drugs of which they know little, to cure diseases on which they know less, into humans of which they know nothing." As our knowledge of the body's role in healing grows, science may look back to nature for help in developing a new generation of medicines in tune with the body's own healing system.

In many areas, medical technology has outpaced our ability to manage its implications humanely. A very premature infant who is tethered by a tube to a mechanical ventilator or an elderly patient who is supported by machines and medicinal chemistry in an intensive care unit may each be as much the victim of modern medicine as its beneficiary. Who should be treated with the new technologies? Who should pay for them? Just because we know how to create babies outside the womb, should we create them? How much should quality of life count in making medical decisions? How do our health and health care relate to who we are as persons? It is little wonder that ethics and economics are among the fastest-growing fields of medical study in the 1990s.

Another cost of scientific medicine has been a gradual change in the age-old relationship between healer and patient. Until about fifty years ago, most patients were treated in the home, and doctors routinely noted in their records such details of a patient's life as employment, living standard, and family circumstance. In this they followed Hippocrates's dictum to "study all these signs and to analyze what they portend." Such treatment is rare today. Patient care has moved from home and family to impersonal hospitals and clinics. As practitioners of Western medicine have become more confident of their skills, they have shifted the emphasis from the patient to diseases, technological diagnosis, and chemically based treatment.

Even the diagnostic tools and techniques doctors use, sometimes to save our lives, have alienated us from our physicians. This alienation began as early as 1819, when the French physician René Laennec introduced a new listening device called the stethoscope. Before then, a doctor who wanted to listen to a patient's heart put his ear on the patient's chest. But the stethoscope made it possible to listen to many bodily sounds, and soon doctors were developing a new diagnostic vocabulary to describe the sounds of the human heart, belly, and lungs. Since then, diagnostic tools and tests have proliferated with ever-increasing sophistication. These include special x-rays, computerized scans, and miniaturized instruments for peering into body cavities; instruments for measuring physiological functions,

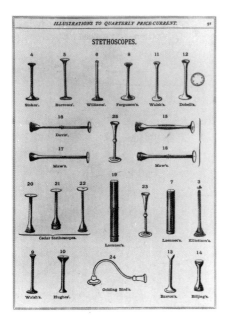

such as lung capacity and the electrical activity of the heart; ever-more-advanced microscopic techniques for visualizing body cells and disease-producing bacteria; and a growing arsenal of specialized laboratory tests.

Doctors have gradually come to rely on such tests over other diagnostic considerations. But although a thousand-dollar computerized scan may tell a physician the exact dimensions of an illness, it cannot reveal what having the illness means to the patient. The patient in such a scheme becomes an object of study, a broken machine. And when the body is seen as a machine, doctors inevitably become mechanics, fixing or replacing parts, chemically readjusting faulty systems. Through the success of this approach, medical science has spawned a vast professional healing class, along with the widespread belief that healing is something doctors do for us, not something we do for ourselves, sometimes with a doctor's help. Our concept of health no longer reflects the root meaning of *whole, wholesome, hallowed,* and *holy.* To be healthy in our culture means to be in good repair, well tuned, firing on all cylinders, to be simply *not* sick.

The development of the stethoscope began a long period in which physical signs and scientific data were the central criteria for establishing diagnosis and treatment. The earliest stethoscopes simply provided a channel for sound between the patient's body and the physician's ear. Above: A catalog illustration from 1869. Right: The development of modern diagnostic technologies has given doctors increasingly detailed information about the physical composition and functioning of the human body. This fluoroscope from the 1930s was a forerunner of the modern x-ray machine.

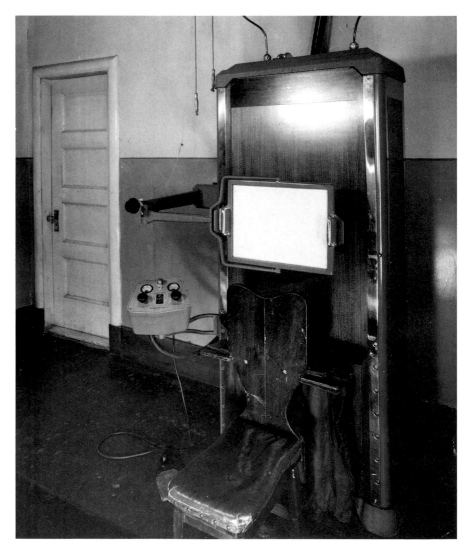

What Causes Disease?

Throughout the development of the Western medical tradition, however, some physicians and others have persistently suggested that medicine might be more complicated than mechanics. Among the earliest contributors to this debate were two late-nineteenth-century giants of French medicine, who argued one of the most-asked questions of all times: What makes people sick? One of these giants was the chemist Louis Pasteur, who changed medical history by linking specific microorganisms to rabies and other human diseases. The other was Claude Bernard, a pioneer physiologist with the heart of a philosopher and an incalculable respect for the complexities of the human body. Their discourse on the cause of disease was central to the life and work of both men—Pasteur was moved to make his final contribution to the discussion virtually at death's door.

The discovery by Pasteur and others that microorganisms are associated with disease was among the earliest successes of scientific medicine. Based on this knowledge, medicine would quickly develop "magic-bullet" treatments for many terrible diseases: a vaccine for tuberculosis, insulin for the management of diabetes, and, after the 1940s, antibiotic cures for many bacterial infections. The observed relationship between microorganisms and disease led to the Theory of Specific Etiology, which held that every disease or infection is caused by a specific microorganism—and, by extension, that all diseases have a single identifiable cause.

But what did it mean to say an organism caused a disease? Did that mean the organism alone could make someone sick? This notion fit well with the emerging model of the body as a machine. Based on this model, the disease came from the outside, as though someone had chucked a handful of sand into a contentedly purring engine. But might not disease also be caused by some weakness in the infected person that allowed the organism to flourish? This concept looked backward to Hippocrates—and looked forward, as well, toward our own growing understanding that disease may spring from a multitude of physical, environmental, cultural, emotional, spiritual, and psychological roots.

Back and forth the debate flourished. Not

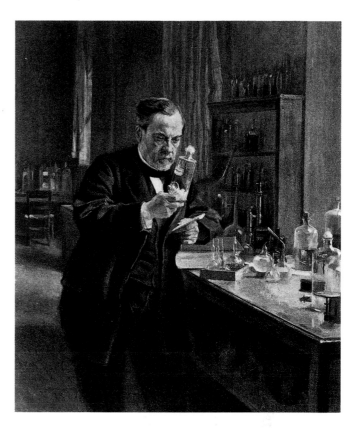

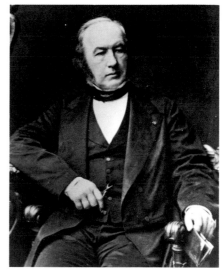

Louis Pasteur (above) emphasized the role of the invading microorganism in causing disease, but Claude Benard (right) believed that the condition of the person infected might be more important in determining whether disease develops.

In recognizing that the mind can affect bodily processes, Western research is merely acknowledging what the practitioners of some Eastern religions have known for centuries. Hindu and Buddhist yogis have long practiced bodily control over such seemingly "automatic" functions as skin temperature, heart rate, and metabolism as an aid to spiritual enlightenment.

As early as the eighteenth century, reports began reaching the West of seemingly impossible feats performed by Buddhist and Hindu yogis. In 1837, an Indian yogi named Haridas had himself buried alive for six weeks, an event reported on by several reliable Western observers. Before the burial Haridas cleansed his stomach with a long strip of cloth and his bowels with enemas and sealed his ears, nostrils, and rectum with wax. He then was placed in a white cloth bag, locked in a wooden box, and placed in a subterranean chamber surrounded by a large building.

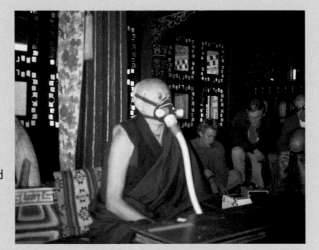

To forestall accusations of fraud, Haridas asked the local maharaja to supervise his interment and to maintain a constant guard over the building, which was also padlocked and sealed with the maharaja's seal. Sir Claude Wade, a local British official, accompanied the maharaja when the seal was broken six weeks later and the wooden box unlocked and the yogi lifted into the room.

The cloth bag enclosing the yogi appeared mildewed, Wade reported, as though it had been buried for some time. "The legs and arms of the body were shriveled and stiff, the face full, the head reclining on the shoulder like that of a corpse." Wade called for a doctor, who "could discover no pulsation in the heart, the temples, or the arm. There was, however, a heat about the region of the brain, which no other part of the body exhibited."

Wade then describes how the yogi's servant bathed the body in warm water, cleared the nostrils and ears, and gradually resuscitated Haridas from a state like hibernation in which he seemed very close to death. Within half an hour, Haridas was talking feebly. "We then left him," Wade wrote, "convinced that there had been no fraud or collusion in the exhibition we had witnessed."

As electronic monitoring devices became available in the twentieth century, researchers crisscrossed India trying to measure yogic accomplishments more concretely. Many yogis showed impressive control over heart rate, respiration, skin conductance, and skin temperature. One finding, which might explain in part how yogis are able to undergo a living burial, showed that some yogis could reduce their metabolism to use less oxygen.

One of the most thoroughly studied yogic abilities is also one of the most dramatic. In 1979, Harvard cardiologist Herbert Benson, who had researched the physical effects of Eastern meditation, sought permission to study g Tummo ("heat") yoga, in which experienced Tibetan Buddhist monks warm their near-naked bodies through meditation, even in freezing temperatures.

It is important to understand what an unlikely accomplishment this is. Mammals maintain body heat in cold weather by growing fur coats or, in the case of humans, putting on more clothes. If the body remains cold after these

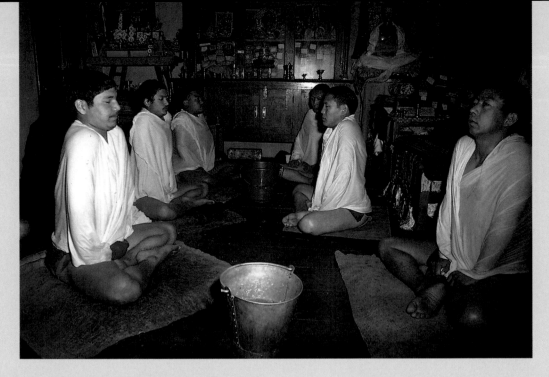

Dr. Benson documented the meditation of Tibetan Buddhist monks. Opposite page: A monk decreases his metabolism, from rest, 64 percent. This is the greatest reduction in energy consumption, from rest, ever recorded in humans. This page: Monks perform *g Tummo* yoga.

precautions, bodily reflexes take over. The muscles begin to shiver involuntarily to produce extra heat. At the same time, the blood vessels of the skin constrict, so less heat is lost through the circulating blood, preserving warmth for the heart, lungs, kidneys, and other organs in the body interior. The *g Tummo* monks were said to abort this automatic process. They did not shiver, and their skin stayed warm. Perhaps they were able to increase their metabolism somehow, generating more heat. Or perhaps they were shifting body heat to the surface by controlling the constriction and dilation of their peripheral blood vessels.

Western scientists had never before been allowed to study the monks. But Benson sought and received permission to do so from the Dalai Lama of Tibet. Several times over the next few years, he and his researchers traveled to the Indian town of Upper Dharmsala, the Dalai Lama's home base. From there they would hike into the Himalayan foothills surrounding the town, where the monks lived in isolated, unheated stone huts at six to seven thousand feet above sea level.

One day, Benson watched the monks wrap their bodies in soaking-wet sheets. The room temperature was approximately 40° Fahrenheit, and the water measured approximately 49°. Under such conditions the human body is programmed to begin shivering uncontrollably.

But within five minutes the meditating monks were generating enough body heat that the sheets began to steam, fogging the lenses of the researchers' cameras. Within half an hour the sheets were completely dry. The monks repeated the exercise twice more.

On another night a group of monks meditated for eight hours outdoors at nineteen thousand feet above sea level while the temperature was 0° and snow fell. In the morning the monks shook off the snow and walked back to their monastery, two thousand feet down the hill. When asked how they performed such feats, the monks speak of an inner heat ignited through the gathering of a natural energy, called *prana*, a word literally meaning "wind" or "air." Of course, Benson had no way of measuring *prana* or the religious discipline that enabled the monks to exhibit such impressive bodily control. He could, however, document the control and suggest what physiological processes might be involved. He measured heart rates and the temperature at ten different spots on the bodies of meditating monks. With room temperatures hovering around 40°, the nearly-naked monks were able to warm their fingers and toes by as much as fourteen degrees. The most likely reason for the increase in temperature, Benson concluded, was an extraordinary ability to control blood flow to vessels of the skin.

surprisingly, Pasteur, the pioneer microbiologist, was inclined to believe that microbes were the most important factor in infectious disease. But Bernard, the physiologist who had begun to unravel the intricacies of the liver and pancreas, was impressed by the body's ability to adjust, to maintain internal balance. He spoke of the *milieu interieur*, the "inner environment," and of *le terrain*, literally translated "the soil." The microbe was like a seed, Bernard said, that would sprout into disease only if the "soil" or internal environment were too weak to resist.

Our modern knowledge of the role of the immune system in preventing disease has confirmed that Bernard was right. We now understand that whether or not somebody gets an infection depends on many factors, including the strength of the microbe, the number of microbes that invade, as well as Bernard's *milieu interieur*. We know that when our resistance is low, we may be unable to resist a cold or flu virus that otherwise would not make us sick.

It is now clear also that microorganisms alone cannot make us sick. The Epstein-Barr virus, for example, is associated with numerous diseases, including infectious mononucleosis, certain cancers of the nose and pharynx, and Burkitt's lymphoma, a malignant tumor of children. Yet many people carry the virus and never get any of the illnesses associated with it. Why do some people get one illness from the virus rather than another? We don't know, but it seems that the virus alone does not cause any one of these diseases. Similarly, not every person infected with the human immunodeficiency virus (HIV) inevitably comes down with AIDS, the deadly infection of the immune system with which that virus has been associated. Although HIV is apparently necessary to produce AIDS, it does not always produce AIDS in every person. Of the millions of people infected with HIV, scientists have identified at least seventy people who have been carrying the virus for as long as fourteen years and so far have shown no signs of HIV-related illness. Why do some people succumb quickly to HIV while others live for years without becoming ill? Again, this may have to do with individual differences or perhaps with some as yet unidentified "cofactor" that is necessary to produce the disease.

Despite mounting evidence of its importance, modern medicine has paid relatively little attention to *le terrain*. We have studied extensively the external factors associated with disease—microorganisms, carcinogenic chemicals, and the like—but know relatively little about the inner physical and mental conditions that may predispose that soil for disease.

As for Pasteur, he gradually grew to accept his friend Bernard's views and on his deathbed is said to have made the ultimate concession: "*Bernard avait raison. Le germe n'est rien, c'est le terrain qui est tout.*" ("Bernard was right. The germ is nothing; the soil is everything.") This was an overreaction, of course—the germ is clearly not nothing. But it is not everything either.

Diseases from the Unconscious

At about the same time that Pasteur and Bernard were arguing the subtleties of infectious disease, a neurologist named Jean Martin Charcot was demonstrating through hypnosis that some diseases clearly arose from deep within the *milieu interieur*. A century after Franz Mesmer had been drummed out of Parisian society for practicing what would come to be known as hypnosis, Charcot was giving the process new legitimacy in a series of dramatic public lectures. No wild-eyed arm-flapper in a lilac gown, Charcot was known as the Napoleon of Neurology, and he attracted students from across Europe. In one crowd-pleasing experiment Charcot would hypnotize a patient suffering from supposedly irreversible paralysis. He would then command the patient to rise and walk before the eyes of the amazed audience. When Charcot withdrew the hypnotic suggestion, the patient would collapse on the stage at his feet, leaving no doubt that the patient's very real incapacity extended from some unlit corner of the mind.

On some level humankind has probably always known about what we now call the "unconscious," that part of the mind of which we are not aware. Every shaman entering a trance, every priest of Asclepios interpreting a patient's dream, was essentially courting the unconscious realm. In his magnetizing trances, Mesmer dramatically introduced the unconscious to the rationalistic world of Western medicine. But it was not until Charcot's time that

Western science began to speculate formally on the powers of the unconscious, using hypnosis as a tool.

In his lectures, Charcot discussed hysterical illness, in which a physical symptom—paralysis, for example—seems to arise from some psychological, often unconscious, cause. Also in the 1880s, Pierre Janet, another French researcher, began speculating on dissociation, a kind of "block" between the conscious and unconscious that could be overcome through hypnosis. And taking it all in from a seat in Charcot's and Janet's lecture halls was the man who would become the high priest of the unconscious, a visiting Viennese psychiatrist named Sigmund Freud. His influence on our culture has been so profound that the vocabulary of the unconscious joined the language of the streets. Most of us understand, for example, that to *repress* a painful thought, memory, or emotion means to push it out of the conscious realm. Building on Charcot's work, Freud came to believe that unexpressed, chronically repressed emotions might eventually result in physical symptoms or disease.

Over the next decades, while most practitioners of Western medicine were focused on understanding and repairing the machinelike body, psychiatry became the custodian of the ancient idea that the mind can affect physical health. By the 1930s, a Chicago psychiatrist, Dr. Franz Alexander, was laying the groundwork for what would become a whole new field of medicine. "Many chronic disturbances are not caused by external, mechanical, chemical factors, or by microorganisms," Alexander wrote in 1939, "but by the continuous functional stress arising during the everyday life of the organism in its struggle for existence." The new field, called *psychosomatic medicine*, was built on the observations of many medical specialists that certain conditions seemed particularly associated with emotional upset. Nothing brought this home as clearly as the turmoil of World War II. Suddenly, military doctors were reporting case after case of what Dr. Alexander referred to as *organ neuroses*—emotionally triggered disturbances of the stomach, bowels, or heart. Many doctors looked at these diseases as somehow suspect, not as real as diseases from bugs, bullets, or other physical causes.

By the 1950s, a list of seven core psychosomatic ailments had been developed—diseases thought to be worsened by psychological stress. Among these ailments were warts and other diseases of the skin. Asthma, stomach ulcers, and ulcerative colitis (an

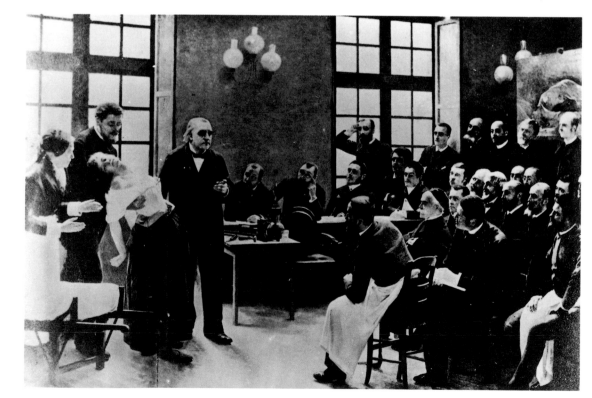

Jean Martin Charcot, who brought respectability to hypnosis and the influence of mind on disease, demonstrates how hypnosis can affect the symptoms of an "hysterical" disease.

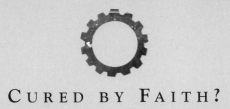

CURED BY FAITH?

On May 4, 1947, a former foundry worker named George Orr attended a Christian healing service near Pittsburgh, Pennsylvania. Twenty-two years earlier, Orr had been splashed in the right eye with molten iron. Nearly blinded by the burn, he had been examined by Dr. C. E. Imbrie and was granted full compensation for permanent disability by the Pennsylvania Department of Labor and Industry.

Presiding at the service that day was Kathryn Kuhlman, who would become one of twentieth-century America's best-known faith healers. Born about 1915, Kuhlman began her career as a Christian evangelist. She apparently began faith healing in 1946, after a man at one of her services announced that his tumor had disappeared following a service led by Kuhlman the preceding day.

During the 1960s and 1970s, Kuhlman's healing services would regularly fill the huge Shrine Auditorium in Los Angeles.

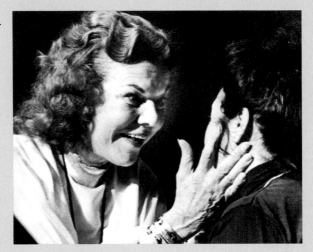

After an emotionally charged warm-up of hymn singing, Kuhlman would stride onto the stage and begin to preach. She talked of God's love — for which she claimed to be only a conduit — and, after intensive prayers, would begin to point to areas of the auditorium where she intuited that a healing was taking place. Soon people would rise, one by one, to testify that they had been healed.

George Orr did not rise to testify on that May day in 1947. But standing beside his wife during the service, he suddenly became convinced that spiritual healing was possible. Later he would report that he had begun to pray and had almost immediately experienced a tingling in his damaged eye, accompanied by an uncontrollable flow of tears. In the car after the service, Orr discovered he could see perfectly, and he would soon learn that the scar on his eye had completely disappeared. Dr. Imbrie, who examined the eye two years later, was reportedly astonished at the healing.

This story was reported by Allen Spraggett, a former Christian minister and reporter for the *Toronto Star,* who became interested in parapsychology and investigated some of Kuhlman's healings in the 1960s. Among the other cases Spraggett related was that of Karen George, a baby with a clubfoot and a twisted leg that began to straighten on the trip home from the healing service and was completely cured within two days.

Other investigators were more critical of Kuhlman's work. In the 1970s, Dr. William Nolen interviewed twenty-three people who claimed to be cured as a result of Kuhlman's healings. He found ample evidence that people felt better but no objective proof of medical cures. Like many critics of faith healing, Nolen came to believe that people simply felt better because they believed they would.

Many Americans associate faith healing with the fundamentalist Christian traditions. But similar healing ceremonies take place in many cultures. Common features include a gathering of emotionally charged people brought to a hypnotic, trancelike state through singing, prayer, chanting, or dance.

In the American South, some Christian groups enhance this emotionalism by handling poisonous snakes, taking as their text a biblical passage from St. Mark: "In my name they shall cast out devils; they shall speak in new tongues; they shall take up serpents; and if they drink

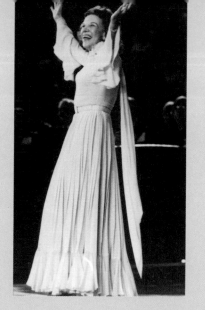

This page: Kathryn Kuhlman leading a "miracle" service in 1975. Opposite page: During a rally in Detroit, Kuhlman touches the cheek of a woman seeking help.

any deadly thing, it shall not hurt them; they shall lay hands upon the sick and they shall get well."

In Zimbabwe, in south-central Africa, white-garbed Christian apostolics gather at huge outdoor healing ceremonies to dance, sing, shout, and court the Holy Spirit. On the beaches of Santos, on the coast near São Paulo, Brazil, up to a quarter of a million adherents of the Afro-Brazilian Umbanda religion gather each New Year's Eve to celebrate the Festival of Iemanja, goddess of the spring, with dancing, singing, and ritual trance.

Detractors liken such gatherings to mass psychodrama. They point out that most of the cures are of diseases known to be particularly sensitive to psychological states. They accuse American faith healers of being charlatans who take unfair advantage of the sick to fill the collection plate and support sophisticated direct-mail, fund-raising schemes.

But many people seem to feel better after the emotional discharge of a faith healing ceremony — and this is itself a kind of healing. In other people, belief, expectation, or trance may work the changes in the body through established placebo mechanisms or other mechanisms we have yet to understand. There can never be any irrefutable proof that the love of God working through Kathryn Kuhlman effected cures in George Orr or the baby Karen George. But we do know that expectant faith, belief, and altered states of mind are associated with many kinds of healing.

inflammation of the large intestine), as well as some forms of high blood pressure, arthritis, and thyroid disease, were also on the list.

Stress: Pioneer Connections

It is hard for us now, sixty years after Western doctors first suggested that stress might play a role in human health, to understand how radical the suggestion seemed at the time. These days it is common to talk about being "stressed out" by the pressures of everyday life. But when Dr. Hans Selye first popularized the term in the 1930s, the idea seemed exotic to physicians who still saw the mind and body as separate entities. Selye was an endocrinologist at the University of Montreal who had been a student of Harvard physiologist Dr. Walter Cannon. Together, the work of Cannon and Selye reintroduced to Western medicine Claude Bernard's concept of the *milieu interieur*. Cannon described a process he called homeostasis, the body's continual attempt to achieve internal balance in response to external change. Selye suggested that if the change was too great, the body might not be able to adjust and disease would result.

In many ways the current interest in the mind-body connection can be traced directly to the work of Dr. Selye and Dr. Cannon, which outlined the actual mechanisms through which the mind might contribute to disease. In Western medicine, understanding how such a process happens is essential to its being accepted as true. Dr. Cannon traced the mechanisms of stress to the *autonomic nervous system*, which regulates such vital functions as heartbeat, blood pressure, and digestion. When a person walks up a hill, for example, the autonomic nervous system signals the heart to beat faster and the lungs to draw in more air. Cannon observed that the body also responds to emotional cues, which is why the heart beats faster when a person is startled, anxious, or sexually aroused. The autonomic nervous system evolved over tens of thousands of years, in part to help the human organism respond to outside dangers. An early human facing a saber-toothed tiger needed to be instantly ready either to run or to stand his ground. When faced with such a danger, the autonomic nervous system directs the heart rate and rate of breathing to increase, raises the blood sugar

Opposite page: The autonomic nervous system, which sends nerves to many organs of the body, consists of two parts. The *sympathetic* branch (represented in the left half of the illustration) is in part responsible for the fight-or-flight response. It increases the heart rate, raises blood pressure, releases sugar from the liver to nourish the muscles, and slows digestion as it shunts blood from the stomach and intestines to the heart and muscles for quick action. The *parasympathetic* branch (represented in the right half of the illustration) has just the opposite effects. It slows heart rate, lowers blood pressure, and moves blood to the stomach and intestines to promote efficient digestion. Long thought to be largely "automatic," the autonomic nervous system is now understood to respond to emotional cues and mental states. The sympathetic branch mediates some of the effects of stress on the body, while mind-body healing techniques, such as meditation, work in part by activating the parasympathetic, slowing branch of the system.

level to supply the body with quick energy, and shunts blood from the digestive system into the large muscles, where it can do the most good. Cannon called this process the *fight-or-flight* mechanism.

Many of the body's responses to stress were chemical, Cannon taught. Under stress, the brain prompts the release of certain fight-or-flight chemicals—neurotransmitters from nerve endings and hormones from certain glands. These "internal drugs" were the first to be recognized in what would become an emerging pharmacy of mind-body chemicals.

Building on Dr. Cannon's work, Dr. Selye formalized the concept of stress and identified what he called the "stress response," a set of physiological reactions to changing physical conditions or emotional upset. His work was critical in showing how emotional distress can lead to disease through chemical mind-body connections. It is these chemical connections that prompt palpitations of the heart, "butterflies" in the stomach, and other symptoms of nervousness and anxiety. Dr. Franz Alexander and other exponents of psychosomatic disease had also recognized the importance of these connections. Diseases linked to emotional causes were now understood (and sometimes misunderstood) to be over- or underresponses of parts of the autonomic nervous system.

This early work on the mind-body link suggested that the human way of life was evolving too fast for the human body to keep up. The fight-or-flight reaction, so helpful in the face of acute danger, could be a liability when the danger was long term and relatively diffuse—when the threat was not an animal in the bushes but persistent grinding fear that one might lose one's job or fail academically or not live up to one's own expectations. The early stress researchers began to develop a framework for understanding how people can "worry themselves sick."

The modern recognition that stress can contribute to disease eventually led to thousands of research studies linking the mind to illness, healing, and bodily states. Gradually, these studies are confirming many ideas about healing common to all cultures: the importance of belief in healing, the healing power of the unconscious, health as an ever-adjusting balance between a multitude of physical, psychological, and spiritual variables. At the same time, the public has become fascinated with the concept of "holistic" (or "wholistic") health—the pursuit of health for the whole person through a variety of mind-body techniques—and this public interest has helped drive scientific research. Today, Dr. Selye and Dr. Cannon are seen as pioneers, among the first researchers to use the tools of Western science to demonstrate that Descartes was wrong—that the mind and the body are indivisible.

"I have always felt that the only trouble with scientific medicine is that it is not scientific enough," wrote twentieth-century microbiologist and philosopher of science René Dubos. "Modern medicine will become really scientific only when physicians and their patients have learned to manage the forces of the body and the mind that operate in *vis medicatrix naturae*"—according to the healing power of nature.

AUTONOMIC NERVOUS SYSTEM

Sympathetic
Nervous
System

Parasympathetic
Nervous
System

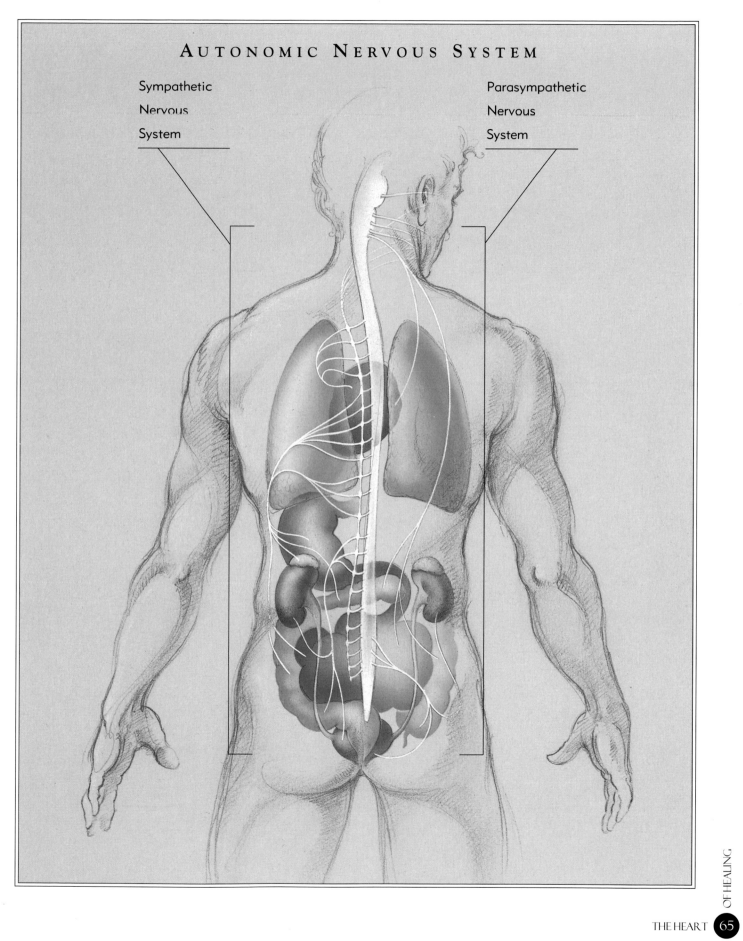

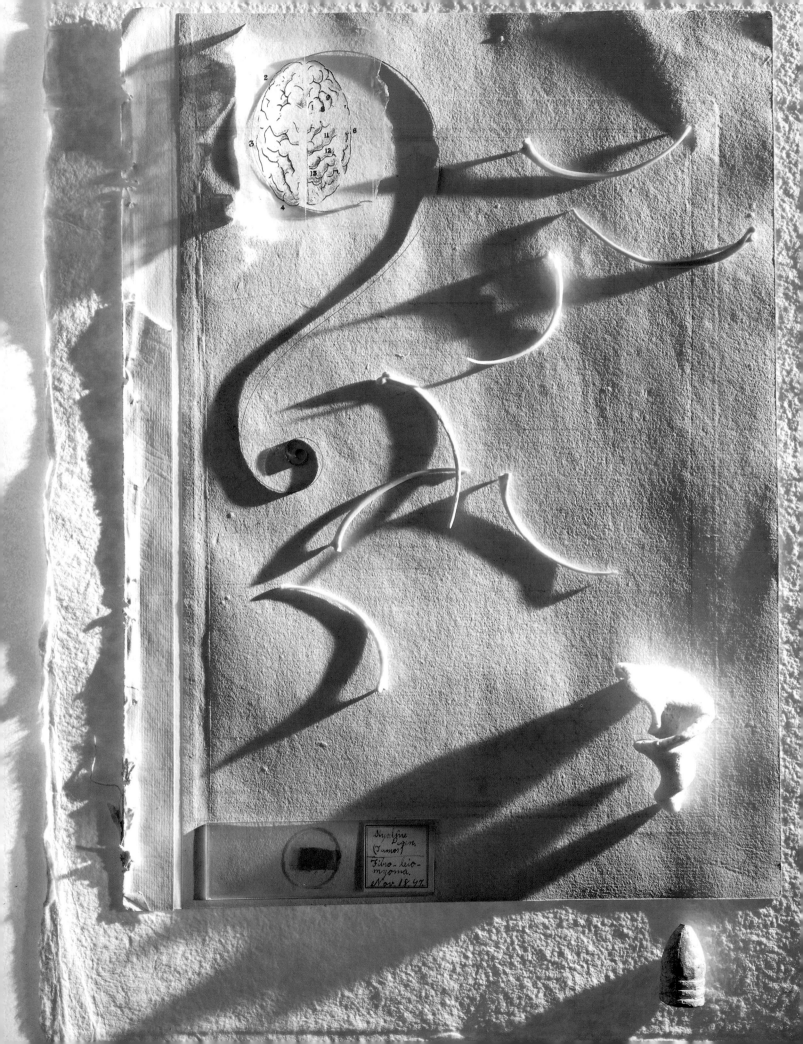

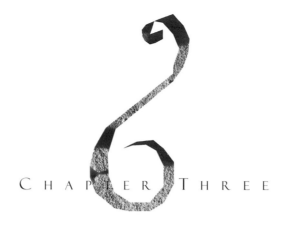

C H A P T E R T H R E E

MIND, BRAIN, AND IMMUNITY

IN SEARCH OF HEALING CONNECTIONS

A S Y S T E M F O R T H E B O D Y ' S H E A L T H

IN THE EARLY 1970S, a young doctor named Carl Simonton raised eyebrows in the American medical community by implying that the mind could help cure cancer. Simonton, who had been trained at the University of Oregon Medical School as a cancer specialist with a subspecialty in radiation, had noticed that a positive attitude seemed to help some patients survive "unsurvivable" disease. When he asked the patients why they thought they were doing so well, he heard answers concerning their wishes and obligations: to see a son or daughter graduate from college, to help co-workers complete a project, to resolve long-standing family problems. The common theme of their replies, Simonton maintained, "was the belief that they *exerted some control over the course of their disease*."

Working closely with his wife, Stephanie, a motivational psychologist, Dr. Simonton began studying biofeedback, group therapy, meditation, motivational training, and several mind-control techniques that were gaining popularity. Gradually, the team emphasized visual imaging, which called for a "focused relaxation" similar to hypnosis during which the person forms a mental picture of a desired goal.

> *"The healing system is the way the body mobilizes all its resources to combat disease. The belief system is often the activator of the healing system."*
>
> —NORMAN COUSINS

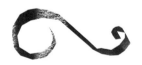

"Concentrate on your cancer," Simonton told the first patient he treated using the technique. The man was sixty-one years old and suffering from throat cancer, for which Dr. Simonton was supervising last-chance radiation treatments. "Picture the radiation as millions of tiny bullets of energy bombarding the cancer cells," he instructed. "Visualize the immune system's white blood cells swarming over the weakened cancer cells. Picture the tumor shrinking and the return of health."

The patient responded beyond the Simontons' most optimistic expectations. Not only did the man's cancer improve, but he used the imaging technique to work on two other long-standing health problems and soon announced that he had cured himself of both arthritis and sexual impotence. Buoyed by this and other successes, the Simontons established the Cancer Counseling and Research Center in Fort Worth, Texas, where patients from across the country have learned to participate in their own healing. (Simonton has since moved his work to the Simonton Cancer Center, in Pacific Palisades, California.) By 1978, when their best-selling book, *Getting Well Again*, was published, the couple claimed to have treated 159 "incurable" cancer patients. All had been told that they would die within a year, but most lived at least twenty months, and about a fourth recovered partially or completely from their disease.

Such reports caught the imagination of the press and the public—the Simontons appeared on television, and their work was featured in newspapers and magazines. To the medical establishment, however, the assertion that attitude could affect cancer was pure quackery. Doctors had learned to be cautious of claims that extraordinary treatments could cure incurable disease. To them, many of the Simontons' ideas were based more on colorful anecdotes than on hard data. Particularly troubling was the implication that the mind could influence the immune system—that by visualizing their white blood cells "devouring" their tumors, patients could somehow effect physical changes in their bodies. Such an idea ran counter to fundamental assumptions about immune function. Although other scientists were revealing that the mind has a role in the autonomic nervous system, the wall between mind and immune system seemed inviolate.

Part of the reason the medical community was so resistant to the Simontons' idea had to do with research history. What we knew about the immune system had been learned largely from laboratory investigations: In test-tube experiments and with microscopes, scientists had watched immune cells attack and devour foreign bacteria without help from either body or mind. The immune system seemed completely autonomous, able to defeat disease on its own.

More than twenty years later we understand that the immune system is not an independent defender against disease but a team player. What we had thought of as our primary defense system is in fact only one part of a complex, interactive, mind-body network dedicated to the preservation

Advances in the science of psychoneuroimmunology depend on our ability to measure human immune function, which sounds easier than it is. Scientists must be sure they are measuring immune function changes that are due to their experiments and not to natural differences in immunity. Within limits, immune response can vary with age, sex, race, and nutrition. It can also vary in the same person from hour to hour; immune response is generally lower about an hour after midnight and highest at about 7:00 A.M.

Moreover, there is no single measure of immune function. If we say a person has a fever of 102° Fahrenheit, we are saying something very exact, based on a commonly accepted measure of body temperature. If we say someone has "suppressed immune function," we are saying something relatively inexact, based on one or more of several possible tests—each of which measures a different aspect of overall immunity. Several tests are used to determine immune function:

• Immune-cell counts may be done by computer or simply by counting the cells under a microscope. Frequently, the total number of lymphocytes is counted. Sometimes special markers, called *monoclonal antibodies*, are added to a blood sample. Since these are known to bind to the surface of certain kinds of cells, they facilitate a differential count of the many cells in the sample. An increase in the number of immune cells usually indicates that the body is mounting a response to infection; a dramatic decrease could signal an immune system failure, such as that produced by AIDS or by certain toxic immunosuppressive drugs.

• Immunoglobulins—among them antibodies released by B-cell lymphocytes in response to an invading organism—can be measured in simple tests on blood and saliva. In general, the more responsive the immune system, the higher the immunoglobulin level. For example, resistance to colds can be increased by the presence of one type of an immunoglobulin called IgA in the saliva. IgA is often used as a marker in studies correlating stress with immune function.

• Pin-prick skin tests measure how strongly and rapidly the immune system reacts to an antigen. Most people have had the test for tuberculosis, in which inactivated tuberculosis bacteria are injected beneath the skin. If the test is positive, signaling exposure to tuberculosis, a raised, red wheal appears on the skin within a few days. This *delayed hypersensitive reaction* indicates that the body recognizes the invader and has mounted an immune response. In the pin-prick test for allergies, an immediate reaction shows that the immune system has mounted a defense against the substance being tested.

• Immune function can also be measured in a test tube. Typically, blood cells are mixed with antigens or special solutions that stimulate immune response. One class of stimulants, called *mitogens*, are naturally occurring plant derivatives that cause the proliferation of certain immune cells. The greater the stimulation of these cells, the greater the immune responsiveness of the individual. Researchers have used this kind of test to measure the response of the immune system to emotional factors, such as grief. Other test-tube tests measure the level of the antibodies in blood or the activity of natural killer cells. This test is frequently used in PNI studies.

IMMUNE CELL FUNCTIONS

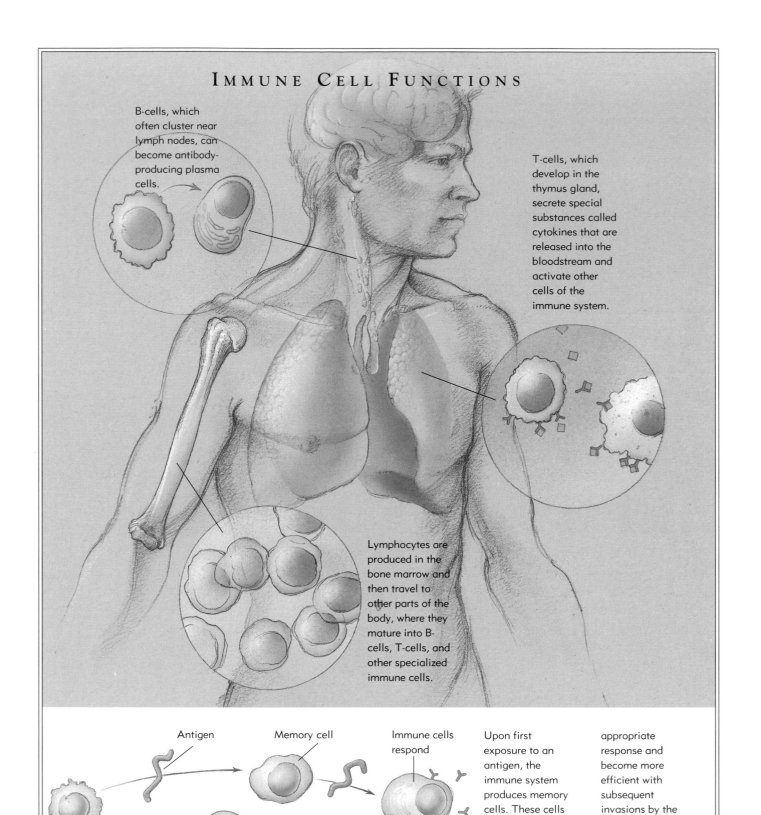

B-cells, which often cluster near lymph nodes, can become antibody-producing plasma cells.

T-cells, which develop in the thymus gland, secrete special substances called cytokines that are released into the bloodstream and activate other cells of the immune system.

Lymphocytes are produced in the bone marrow and then travel to other parts of the body, where they mature into B-cells, T-cells, and other specialized immune cells.

Antigen

Memory cell

Immune cells respond

Immune response becomes more efficient

Upon first exposure to an antigen, the immune system produces memory cells. These cells enable the immune system to remember the appropriate response and become more efficient with subsequent invasions by the microorganism that produces the antigen.

of health. In part, this knowledge has been gained from refined scientific techniques that enable us to study complex biochemical relationships. It has also emerged as a result of a shift in attitude among scientists—a new recognition that mind-body connections might exist, and a new willingness to look for them.

The Department of Defense

The initial discovery in the science of immunology occurred tens of thousands of years ago, probably with the observation that most wounds heal on their own. But it wasn't until the invention of the microscope in the seventeenth century that scientists got a good look at the agents of that process: transparent cells in the blood, which they called white blood cells to differentiate them from the only other identified cells, which were red. White blood cells, early scientists noticed, streamed to the site of an infection or fresh wound. And, as microscopes improved, scientists noticed that some of these cells—later called *phagocytes*—engulfed and destroyed foreign particles in the blood. This and similar discoveries led to the most popular metaphor for the immune system: a defending army protecting the "homeland" of the body against disease. This army assumes two strategies for defense. During *cell-mediated* immunity, specialized blood cells alert the immune system to invaders—particularly viruses and tumors—and organize a direct response by the cells. *Humoral immunity*, more often active against bacteria, depends on special molecules in body fluids. Some of these molecules, called *antibodies*, are released by immune cells when they detect the presence of molecular *antigens* from invading organisms.

One crucial group of immune cells—called *lymphocytes*—are manufactured in bone marrow, the porous inner spaces of the body's long bones. Then, like soldiers leaving boot camp, many stream to other organs for specialized training. About half the lymphocytes are trained in the thymus gland, a walnut-sized organ behind the breastbone, and so are called *T-cell lymphocytes*, or simply *T-cells*. Other lymphocytes, called *B-cells*, cluster near lymph nodes, where they produce antibodies active against disease.

Specialized lymphocytes include *suppressor T-cells* and *helper T-cells*, which help regulate the immune response, and *killer T-cells*, which take aim at invaders. Other specialized immune cells include *monocytes* and *macrophages* (both phagocytes) and *NK* (or *natural killer*) *cells*, which are particularly active against tumors. In the time it has taken you to read the last few paragraphs your body has produced about 10 million new lymphocytes and a million billion new antibody molecules.

But as impressive as this disease-fighting arsenal may seem, the real power of the immune system comes from its command and control of immune function. To fight disease and preserve health, the immune system must excel at the "three Rs." It must *recognize* foreign microorganisms or cancerous cells as distinct from the body's own healthy

Opposite page: Like an army protecting the "homeland," the immune system (top) protects the body from viruses, bacteria, fungi, and cancer cells. Specialized white blood cells called lymphocytes are manufactured in the bone marrow and are released throughout the body. Specialized lymphocytes called B-cells cluster near lymph nodes, where they produce antibodies against potentially harmful microorganisms. T-cell lymphocytes, which develop in the thymus gland, are especially important in organizing immune response. To function properly, the immune system must recognize and react to invaders. In one process central to immune memory (bottom), a B-cell recognizes an antigen released by a microorganism as "foreign." The B-cell can then transform into either a memory cell, which remembers how to defend against the organism, or into a plasma cell, which releases antibodies to fight the invaders.

During the forty years that scientists have been refining our view of the immune system, other researchers have become sophisticated at studying the effects of stress on immunity and disease. In one series of studies, recently reported by Dr. Sheldon Cohen, British volunteers from all walks of life agreed to expose themselves to the common cold virus—delivered through a nasal spray—to see who would get sick. Volunteers were interviewed and filled out a questionnaire about recent life experiences. The researchers found subjects judged to have been under stress before the study were more than twice as likely to come down with colds as those who were not.

An earlier study, in 1979, focused on infectious mononucleosis in West Point cadets. Mononucleosis is one of several diseases associated with a common virus known as the Epstein-Barr (E-B) virus. By adulthood, 85 to 90 percent of Americans have been exposed to the virus and have developed antibodies against it, although only a fraction of that number get

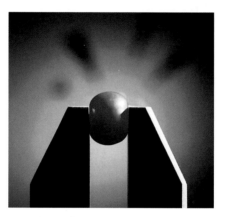

sick from it. At West Point, researchers screened an entire entering class to find those who had never been exposed to the virus. During the next four years, blood was drawn regularly from these unexposed cadets. Each year approximately one-fifth became infected with the E-B virus, but only 25 percent of those who were infected actually contracted the disease.

The researchers also studied West Point's files on each student's family background and academic expectations, and they followed the students' grades and performance. From this research they discovered that students who actually came down with mononucleosis were more likely to have "overachieving" fathers and more likely to be highly motivated for a military career. They were also likely to have poor academic performance. This combination comprised a psychological pincers almost guaranteed to produce high stress.

Herpes viruses such as Epstein-Barr offer a helpful model for studying the effects of stress on immunity: the viruses are very common, and, unlike some other viruses, herpes viruses are never completely wiped out by the immune system but simply are held in check by immune response. Diseases caused by herpes viruses often come and go as the virus advances and retreats. Specific herpes viruses are responsible for recurring oral cold sores and genital ulcers, as well as for chicken pox, and for its recurring form, known as shingles.

The activity of herpes viruses in the body provides a rough measure of the effectiveness of the immune system in holding them back. Researchers can judge this reaction by measuring antibodies to the virus in a person's blood. Having more herpes antibodies, or lower immunity, has been associated with many kinds of stress. Students showed more herpes antibodies while undergoing exams than they did after summer vacation. Divorced and separated men and women showed more antibodies than a matched group of married persons. And psychiatric in-patients showed more antibodies than a matched group of subjects that was not being treated for psychiatric disease.

The same association between stress and herpes holds true for the actual occurrence of disease. In one study, researchers from the University of Pennsylvania and Veterans Administration Hospital in Philadelphia found that typically unhappy people experienced more cold sores than happier subjects. The same group of researchers also found a higher rate of cold sores in students facing exams. In another study, psychologist Margaret Kemeny found that among a group of thirty-six people suffering from the genital form of herpes, depressed individuals experienced more frequent recurrence of the disease. This research provides strong evidence once more that microorganisms alone do not cause infectious disease—that the condition of the person exposed to the microorganism also matters. Scientists are studying, more exactly, how various degrees and duration of stress might affect the immune systems of people at different stages of life and, in turn, how these immune changes might affect health and disease. This will be a much more complicated and long-term task than simply showing that stress and disease are in some way related. Hundreds of these studies have been published.

Much research in this area has been done by Dr. Janice Kiecolt-Glaser, a psychologist, and Dr. Ronald Glaser, an immunology researcher, at the University of Ohio. This husband-and-wife team began researching stress and immune function in the early 1980s and since has studied the immune effects of stresses ranging from marital spats to caring for incapacitated relatives. As an early model for everyday stress, the team selected medical students undergoing exams. For one study, they placed a catheter in one arm of each student and sampled blood for two twenty-four-hour periods—both when students were taking exams and when they were not. Nurses waited outside the students' classrooms to draw blood samples, and the students slept overnight in the health center so regular samples could be drawn. This and other studies show that exams produce an increase in body stress hormones and a decrease in immune function, including a decrease in NK cells, which fight viruses and tumors. This kind of stress is not unique to students, the Glasers believe. Many activities in everyday life involve similar amounts of time pressure and anxiety. Anyone facing a business or tax deadline might

be expected to experience similar stress, along with an increase in bodily stress chemicals and a decrease in immune response.

What is the practical effect of such a decrease on susceptibility to disease? That probably depends on who you are, how you react to stress, how healthy your immune system is, and how long the stress lasts. The Glasers found that, in general, decreased immune function did not lead to increased disease in medical students, perhaps because the subjects were young, had healthy immune systems, and were undergoing short-term stress.

The Glasers began to wonder what would happen if the stress lasted longer and if a person's immune system was not so young and resilient. For a study published in 1991, the Glasers studied sixty-nine persons who had been caring for a spouse with Alzheimer's for an average of five years and compared the immune functions of these long-term caregivers with those of a group from the community, matched according to age, sex, and income. As the Glasers might have expected, the caregivers showed a decrease in three different immune measures. Unlike the young medical students, however, the Alzheimer's caregivers also contracted more illnesses than persons in the matched control group—including a higher rate of influenza, which frequently kills older people.

What surprised the Glasers was that the caregivers did not return to normal after the spouse died and the caregiving was over. Not only were they still preoccupied with issues of caregiving—memories, guilt, persistent thoughts and feelings—but their immune systems also stayed depressed. The Glasers noticed that some caregivers did better than others. Not surprisingly, the key factor in resilience seemed to be strong social support and personal relationships. The caregivers who could turn for relief to others—to family, to friends—were best able to maintain immunity in the face of their unremitting stress.

cells and tissues. It must *remember* what invaders it has previously encountered and how it built a defense against them. Finally, it must *react* with an appropriate response to the threat.

If the immune system is unable to perform any of these tasks, disease can result. In *allergic conditions*, for example, the body misidentifies harmless substances as dangerous and overreacts. The stuffy nose, runny eyes, and other allergic symptoms some people suffer each spring result from an overreaction of the immune system to pollens and other environmental allergens. Similarly, *autoimmune diseases* occur when the immune system misidentifies a part of its own body as an invader and mounts an offensive. Autoimmune diseases include certain forms of diabetes and arthritis and other conditions in which the immune system assaults the body's own joints, muscles, tissues, glands, or organs. The immune system can also underreact to threats, perhaps because it fails to recognize or remember them, or simply because it is not strong enough to mount a defense. If the danger comes from outside the body, from a viral or bacterial invader, the result can be death from overwhelming infection. If it comes from within— because the body's own cells have gone out of control—the result can be cancer.

Influences on Immunity

Nothing has so dramatized the indispensability of a healthy immune system as the emergence of AIDS— acquired immune deficiency syndrome. Historically, immune disorders were thought to be incommunicable—until the early 1980s, when people began dying of an immune deficiency transmitted through infected blood and intimate sexual contact. Persons with AIDS were found to be susceptible to a multitude of viruses, bacteria, fungi, and protozoa to which most persons are immune. They are also susceptible to assault from their bodies' own bacteria or from rare, opportunistic cancers, such as Kaposi's sarcoma. AIDS has been associated with HIV, the human immunodeficiency virus, which attacks T-cells. Physicians follow the course of the syndrome by measuring the T-cell count. Of crucial interest are *helper T-cells*, which stimulate antibody response and may also help create immunologic memory. Normally,

a cubic centimeter of human blood contains more than five hundred helper T-cells; in AIDS patients the figure may approach zero.

Other viruses and some drugs also damage the immune system. Cancers can invade the bone marrow, halting the production of crucial immune cells. Chemotherapy, which works by selectively killing fast-growing cancer cells, will also kill fast-growing immune cells, thereby suppressing immune function. In other cases, immunosuppressive drugs are deliberately prescribed to patients receiving a transplanted heart, kidney, or other organ to prevent its rejection as a foreign invader.

Most doctors long assumed that the immune system was insulated from subtler influences—and certainly from any influence as seemingly insubstantial as the power of the mind—but tantalizing hints of the mind's role in immunity began emerging as early as the 1960s. Between 1968 and 1970, doctors at the National Aeronautics and Space Administration measured the immune function in astronauts during flight and found a decrease in immune response during that short, stressful period when a spacecraft reenters the Earth's gravitational field. These were among the first studies to tie immunosuppression to stress.

A few years later, researchers in separate studies on two continents measured a decrease in immune function among recently widowed men and women. These studies grew from the observation that widowers in particular seemed unnaturally likely to die within six months of a spouse's death. For a study published in 1983, Dr. Steven Schleifer, of Mt. Sinai School of Medicine in New York, periodically drew blood and measured immune response in a group of fifteen men who had lost their wives to breast cancer. These men showed a sharp drop in immune potency two months after the wife's death, and some had not completely recovered ten months later.

Much of the earliest laboratory work on mind and immunity was done in the 1950s by Russian scientists, who believed that immune function might be controlled by the hypothalamus, a grape-sized area at the lower front of the brain. The hypothalamus exercises broad control over numerous body processes, including appetite, temperature, and fluid balance. It

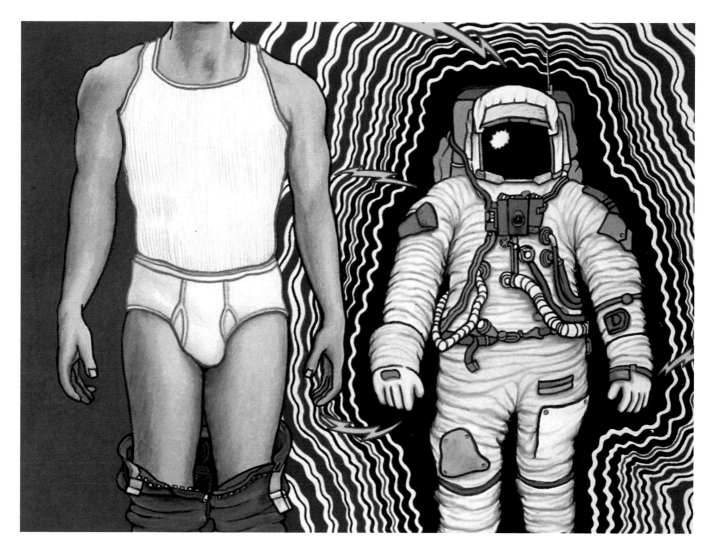

influences the autonomic nervous system and prompts the release of fight-or-flight hormones in times of stress. The hypothalamus is also part of the brain's limbic system, which controls emotion. To prove the link between the hypothalamus and immune function, the Russian researchers destroyed various portions of the hypothalamus in experiments with animals and demonstrated disruption in immune response. It was an intriguing finding—a connection between the hypothalamus and the immune system implied that the immune system might respond to stress and to emotion, too.

In the 1960s, a team of researchers led by psychiatrist George Solomon, who was then at Stanford University, repeated the Russians' studies and launched similar studies of its own. To test whether stress might have an effect on immune response, they introduced tumors into rats and then jolted some of the rats with electric shock. The tumors grew more quickly in the shocked rats, suggesting a decrease in immune response.

Solomon was particularly interested in rheumatoid arthritis and other autoimmune diseases. He had noticed that although several members of

Attitude and Reaction to Disease (above) is "about the onslaught of AIDS," according to artist King Thackston, "and the confusion of that time. It's about the perception of the disease versus how people reacted—your attitude would be one thing, your reaction another." The space suit symbolizes how people removed themselves from physical and emotional contact with anyone with AIDS.

OF HEALING

the same family might carry the genetic factor for rheumatoid arthritis, they did not all suffer the disease's disabling joint pain and deformity. Solomon became convinced that emotions and personality traits must play a role in this overreaction of the immune system to the body's own tissue. In 1965, he published a study comparing the personality traits of female rheumatoid arthritis patients with those of their healthy sisters: The arthritics were found to be more masochistic and self-sacrificing, more compliant and inclined to depression, more likely to deny hostility, and more sensitive to anger. This suggested to Solomon that personality factors and stress played a role in autoimmune disease and therefore that they somehow affected the action of the immune system. Based on what he and others were learning about mind and immunity, Solomon coined a name for the emerging field: *psychoimmunology*.

The Conditioned Immune System

In 1974, one of the central discoveries of mind-body science emerged from a mystery about dying rats. Robert Ader, a psychologist at the University of Rochester, had launched a routine experiment similar to the one made famous by the Russian researcher Ivan Pavlov, who had taught dogs to salivate at the sound of a bell by first associating that sound with the availability of meat. This process of pairing one stimulus (the meat) with a second stimulus (the bell) until the second stimulus alone produced the same result as the first came to be called *behavioral conditioning*. Ader wanted to know how long a conditioned response in rats would last. On the first day of his study, Ader conditioned a group of rats to associate nausea with sugar water by injecting them with a nausea-producing drug just before giving them the sugar water. Each day thereafter he offered the rats sugar water and measured how much they would drink, or how long it would take them to "forget" that the sugar water had once been associated with nausea. On the forty-fifth day, for no apparent reason, some of the rats began to die.

Ader was puzzled. The rats were healthy, young, and well fed. As the researcher reviewed his data, however, a pattern began to emerge. The rats that had died seemed to be the same ones that had drunk the most sugar water. How could that be, since the liquid itself was harmless? Ader reached the startling conclusion that it was not the sugar water that had killed the rats but what they "believed" about the sugar water.

The key to this discovery was the nausea-producing drug Ader had given the rats, cyclophosphamide, also called Cytoxan, which is commonly used for cancer chemotherapy. This drug, a powerful immunosuppressant, is also given to some organ-transplant patients to prevent their immune systems from rejecting transplanted organs. The conditioning had killed the rats, Ader decided. The rats had come to associate the sugar water with nausea, but they had also come to associate the sugar water with immunosuppression, which was why the rats that drank the most sugar water died. With each drink, the rat "believed" it was getting more of the drug and, consequently, its immune system began to fail.

Teaming up with University of Rochester immunologist Nicholas Cohen in the early 1970s, Ader launched a series of experiments to clarify these findings. In one experiment after another, Ader, Cohen, and other researchers demonstrated that the immune response could be either suppressed or enhanced through behavioral conditioning techniques. Somehow the animals' expectations alone seemed to alter their immunity. This response is much like that of people given placebos. In both cases a substance that is supposed to have no physical effect causes changes in the body because the substance becomes associated with other stimuli or events. Ader proposed that, in fact, behavioral conditioning was one way placebos might work. A patient may respond to a sugar pill for the same reason Pavlov's dogs salivated at the sound of a bell, even though the meat had long since disappeared: because the subject somehow "believes" that the stimulus is the real thing.

Following his early experiments, Ader began reviewing other mind-body research. He edited a book, published in 1981, that included articles by major mind-body researchers, which would all but overturn the notion of the independent immune system. In search of a title for the book, Ader considered Solomon's "psychoimmunology" but

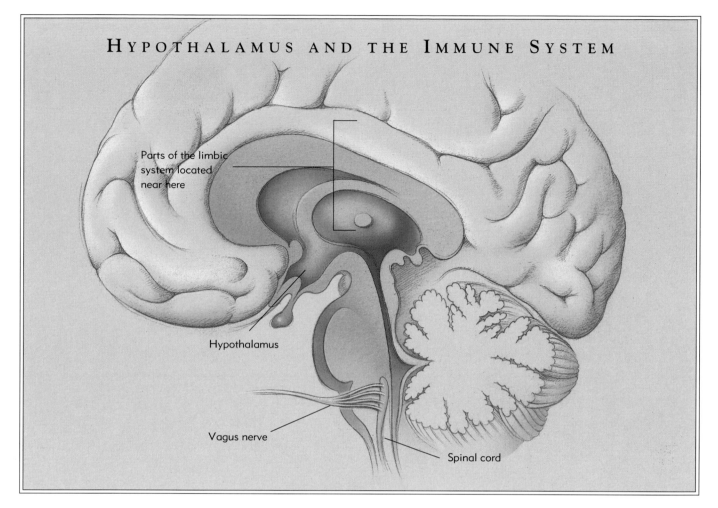

HYPOTHALAMUS AND THE IMMUNE SYSTEM

Parts of the limbic system located near here

Hypothalamus

Vagus nerve

Spinal cord

decided it was important to convey the role of the nervous system. Ader therefore entitled his book *Psychoneuroimmunology*—a new name for a maturing scientific endeavor and a fresh way of thinking about mind, body, and health.

The Inner Language of Immunity

It was one thing for researchers to show there was a relationship between mind and immunity but quite another to demonstrate how that relationship might work. Modern science is often preoccupied with the "how" question, and the ultimate acceptance of psychoneuroimmunology would depend on uncovering its inner mechanisms and connections. It was gradually being established that the mind and immune system somehow communicated with one another, but where did they connect? How did they talk? What languages did they speak?

The logical place to look for connections was the central nervous system—the brain and its vast network of nerves—since research findings linking the brain to immunity were accumulating. Research had shown that damage to the hypothalamus and other portions of the brain could alter immune response. This suggested that messages helping to control immune function flowed from the brain to the body.

Scientists are discovering close relationships between portions of the brain that regulate body function and those associated with thought and emotion. The hypothalamus, shown here in a cross-section through the center of the brain, helps regulate many body functions long thought to be "automatic," such as body temperature. But these functions may, in turn, be influenced by hypothalmic nerve tracks that are part of the limbic system of the brain, which helps regulate emotion, and by other nerve tracks that extend from the hypothalamus into the cerebral cortex, the brain's "thinking cap." Shown also is the vagus nerve, one ot twelve nerves wired directly to the brain, portions of which have recently been traced to the thymus, part of the immune system.

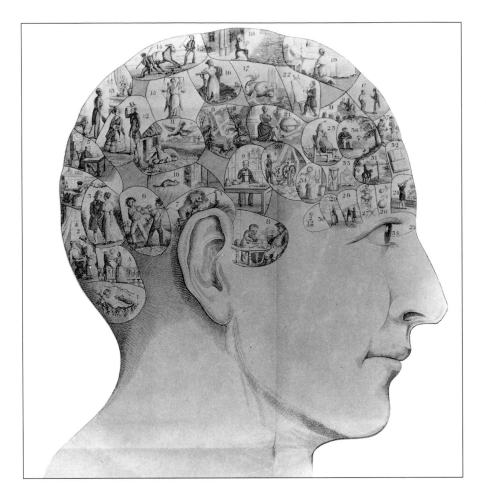

In the West we like to think of science as an ever-growing body of truth. But sciences come and sciences go. In the late 1700s, the science of phrenology postulated that personality could be "read" by feeling the bumps on a person's head. This chart offered a key for the aspiring phrenologist. Notice how bumps indicating such baser tendencies as combativeness, secretiveness, destructiveness, and gluttony are clustered low on the head around the ears.

In the mid-1970s, a Swiss researcher named Hugo Besedovsky studied messages that were transmitted in the other direction, from the immune system to the brain. Besedovsky placed tiny electrodes in the hypothalamus of a rat and measured electrical activity after the animal was injected with powerful antigens. As the rat's body mobilized cells and antibodies to fight the perceived threat, activity in the hypothalamus increased by more than 100 percent—somehow the brain had gotten word that the immune battle was going on.

But how were such messages conveyed? One pivotal finding in the early 1980s was that the organs in the immune system are themselves amply supplied with nerves. Neuroanatomist Karen Bulloch discovered that the thymus, where T-cells are trained to control many immune functions, is infiltrated with branches of the vagus nerve, one of twelve nerves wired directly to the brain. Subsequently, researcher David Felten and a team from the University of Rochester used special fluorescent dyes to trace nerves to the spleen, the lymph nodes, and bone marrow, where most white blood cells are produced. Felten's team discovered a network of nerves near blood vessels that may actually control the flow of lymphocytes through the body. The researchers also showed that the nerves in the thymus and spleen end near clusters of *mast cells*, special cells rich in chemicals that may help control immune function.

Biochemical Messengers

As important as such nerve connections may be, they are only part of an infinitely complex communication system between the brain and the immune system. Much of this dialogue depends on a constant flow of biochemical messages between the two systems, since the immune cells themselves are too mobile for "hard-wired" communications. For such a system to work, and to identify which messages are intended for them, the immune cells recognize the molecular shapes of the biochemical messengers. Each messenger carries a specific combination of molecules that fits a receptor

A Case for Cod Liver Oil

Almost fifteen years after Robert Ader first demonstrated that immune response could be conditioned in rats, he was able to test his approach on a human. The case involved a thirteen-year-old Cleveland girl suffering from lupus erythematosus, a serious autoimmune disease that can affect every part of the body. Because her immune system was attacking her own tissues, the girl had been in and out of the hospital for three years with kidney inflammation, high blood pressure, seizures, and episodes of bleeding. Her bleeding was so serious her doctors had considered a hysterectomy, removal of her womb, out of fear that she she might literally bleed to death when she started menstruating.

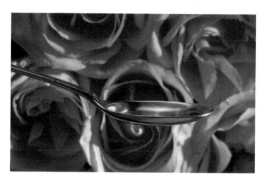

The girl had been treated with blood pressure drugs, antiseizure drugs, diuretics, and steroid hormones to decrease the immune response and inflammation. Now her doctors wanted to launch a major assault against the immune system in hopes of controlling the girl's disease, especially her bleeding. The drug they chose was Cytoxan—the same drug Robert Ader had used to produce immunosuppression in rats. The girl's mother was a psychologist and familiar with Ader's work. She knew the Cytoxan might regulate her daughter's overactive immune system, but she also knew that the drug could be highly toxic. If Ader could condition rats to achieve immunosuppression with low doses of Cytoxan, could he not do the same for her daughter?

Ader was called in by Dr. Karen Olness, the girl's pediatrician. In place of the sugar water used in the rat experiments, Ader and Olness wanted to use a taste that would be "somewhat unpleasant, unforgettable, and previously unknown to the patient." They finally settled on cod liver oil. They also decided to pair a second conditioning stimulus with the drug and chose the unmistakable scent of a strong rose perfume. Once a month, for three months, the girl received intravenous Cytoxan while sipping cod liver oil and then smelling her rose perfume. At the same time, the girl called up the image of a rose in her mind. In the fourth month when she would have ordinarily received the drug, the girl simply drank the oily liquid, uncapped the perfume, and imagined the rose. The treatment lasted a year. Every third month she would receive the drug again, so at the end of a year she had received only six doses when she would have ordinarily received twelve. During the treatments, Ader had good reason to remember that he had originally given Cytoxan to rats to produce nausea. The girl experienced nausea after her very first dose of the drug, and after the third month she could not sip the cod liver oil without retching. Ader decided the nausea might be a conditioned response.

At the end of the treatments, Ader and Dr. Olness concluded that they "seemed as successful as might be expected from a full-dose regimen of the drug." The cod liver oil made her so nauseated she stopped taking it three months after her last dose of Cytoxan. Over the next three years the girl's illness stabilized; her steroid dose was reduced and her blood pressure drug eliminated. Her bleeding problem seemed under control, and she did well in her first year of college. Today, when she wants to call up the drug's immunosuppressive effects, she will still imagine a rose.

Ader and Dr. Olness admitted that no conclusion could be drawn from a single case—especially a case of lupus, which can have a naturally up-and-down course—but they believed other lupus patients might be able to reduce their dose of the dangerous drug.

on the cells much the way a key fits a lock. A messenger can only "unlock" a cell that carries its receptors. This is the mechanism that facilitates the immune system's antigen-antibody response, which is so important in fighting disease. B-cells carry millions of receptor "locks" upon their cell membranes that react with "key molecules" on antigens released by bacteria and other invaders. When the cell encounters an antigen it recognizes, it begins to multiply and to produce antibodies specifically targeted at the invader. This system is so efficient that the body is constantly recognizing and destroying invaders without the person ever feeling sick.

Among the first mind-body messengers to be discovered were *hormones*, which are released by internal glands to help regulate the activity of organs and tissues. Dr. Walter Cannon and Dr. Hans Selye showed how chain reactions of hormones combined with direct nervous stimulation to "turn up" the stress response to help the immune system prepare for emergencies and turn it down again when the crisis has passed. Hormones from the adrenal glands—small, fatty-looking organs atop the kidneys—are critical to this reaction. *Corticosteroid* hormones, from the outer portion or *cortex* of the adrenal glands, raise blood-sugar levels and reduce inflammation. But they also suppress immune response—evidence of their role in immune system communication. Corticosteroids also prompt mood changes, especially depression—a hormonal link that may help explain why immune function is often diminished in clinically depressed patients.

The inside, or *medulla*, of the adrenal glands secrete *epinephrine* and *norepinephrine*, the same fight-or-flight chemicals released by portions of the autonomic nervous system. These hormones increase the heart rate and blood pressure and shunt blood to the large muscles in times of stress. They also influence immune function in ways not yet entirely clear. In a 1983 study, Dr. Joan Borysenko of Boston's Beth Israel Hospital injected volunteers with a small amount of epinephrine—the same amount that would be produced if someone startled you from behind—and measured the blood levels of various immune cells. At first the number of lymphocytes increased, but after thirty minutes the overall number had started to

fall. Closer examination showed a marked increase in suppressor T-cells, which decrease immune response.

Another study at Beth Israel Hospital, in cooperation with researchers from Boston University, showed that norepinephrine, epinephrine's companion hormone, did not suppress immune response but actually increased the activity of the large NK (natural killer) cells thought to be active against cancer. Volunteers for the study received enough of the hormone to produce about as much stress as they'd experience if they were stuck in traffic. On average, they showed almost twice the NK cell activity as before.

Such differing results from similar hormones suggest the immense complexity of the body's chemical control system and the difficulty in pointing to one specific chemical messenger as the consistent "cause" of any single change in immune response. The bloodstream is constantly flooded with a cascade of chemicals, each of which may help modify the action of the others. More than thirty hormones and neurotransmitters have been identified as part of the body's response to stress, and undoubtedly more will be discovered.

The New Messengers of Immunity
Although scientists have long assumed that a receptor mechanism must be responsible for the specificity of biochemical reactions, they have learned only recently how to study the receptors themselves. Some of the most intriguing insights into mind-body communication have emerged from these studies. For example, in the early 1970s, a receptor for morphine and other drugs derived from the opium poppy was identified by Solomon Snyder, of Johns Hopkins University, and a doctoral student, Candace Pert, who would become one of the primary theorists of the new mind-body science. The search for this receptor grew out of the quest for new ways to fight drug addiction. Scientists had thought that drug receptors might be present in the brain—how else would drugs "unlock" the cells to accomplish their work?—but nobody had found a way to test this hypothesis. After trial and error, Pert found a way to prove that the receptors exist by measuring the absorption of a radioactively tagged drug by animal brain tissue.

RECEPTOR MECHANISMS

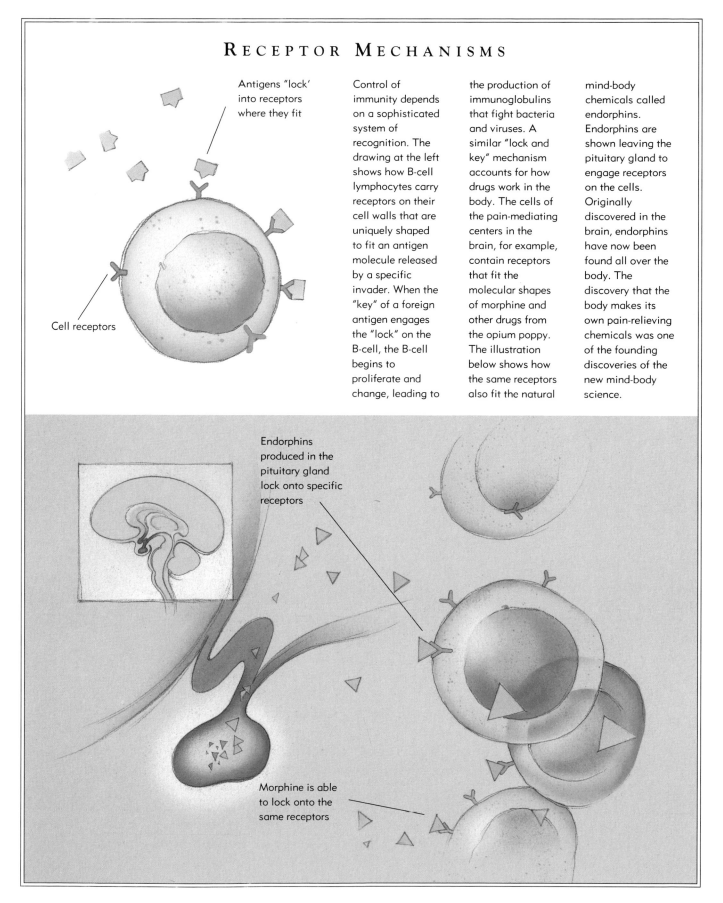

Antigens "lock' into receptors where they fit

Cell receptors

Control of immunity depends on a sophisticated system of recognition. The drawing at the left shows how B-cell lymphocytes carry receptors on their cell walls that are uniquely shaped to fit an antigen molecule released by a specific invader. When the "key" of a foreign antigen engages the "lock" on the B-cell, the B-cell begins to proliferate and change, leading to the production of immunoglobulins that fight bacteria and viruses. A similar "lock and key" mechanism accounts for how drugs work in the body. The cells of the pain-mediating centers in the brain, for example, contain receptors that fit the molecular shapes of morphine and other drugs from the opium poppy. The illustration below shows how the same receptors also fit the natural mind-body chemicals called endorphins. Endorphins are shown leaving the pituitary gland to engage receptors on the cells. Originally discovered in the brain, endorphins have now been found all over the body. The discovery that the body makes its own pain-relieving chemicals was one of the founding discoveries of the new mind-body science.

Endorphins produced in the pituitary gland lock onto specific receptors

Morphine is able to lock onto the same receptors

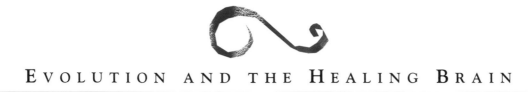

The human brain is the source of much that is marvelous in our lives. Our brains allow us to appreciate the elegance of art, music, literature, mathematics, and philosophy, and to communicate with each other in extraordinary ways. From an evolutionary standpoint, however, the human brain—like the brains of other creatures—has one single overriding purpose: to preserve health, well-being, and the reproductive capacity of the species.

It is a basic tenet of evolutionary theory that all organisms embody characteristics of organisms that have gone before. So it is that the brain of humans today is like a rambling house to which rooms have been added, over time, to meet the needs of increasingly complex organisms. Humans evolved from earlier mammals, which evolved from reptiles. Along the way, new brain structures were added, but remnants of the older structures remain.

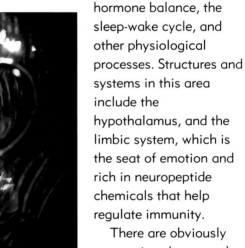

Most of the recent evolutionary development of the human brain has been in the cerebral cortex, sometimes described as the "thinking cap," because it sits atop and is wrapped around older portions of the brain. This structure—which in modern form is about fifty million years old—is largely responsible for sorting information coming in through the senses, for making decisions based on this information and on stored memories, and for sending instructions to other parts of the brain and body. Although the brains of other mammals and reptiles have cortical thinking caps, the development of this region in humans gave the species a remarkable ability to adapt.

The older parts of the brain are most responsible for maintaining life and health—

fulfilling these elementary functions much as they did for our evolutionary antecedents. The deepest, oldest section of the brain is responsible for the most basic coordination of life: breathing, heart rate, and the perceptions that are needed to find prey and avoid predators. Neuroscientist Paul MacLean, who studied the evolution of the brain, calls this the "reptilian" brain because it resembles the brain of present-day reptiles. Somewhat newer but still ancient portions of the brain—what Dr. MacLean calls the "early mammalian brain"—regulate emotion, body temperature, fluid and hormone balance, the sleep-wake cycle, and other physiological processes. Structures and systems in this area include the hypothalamus, and the limbic system, which is the seat of emotion and rich in neuropeptide chemicals that help regulate immunity.

There are obviously connections between the older and younger portions of the brain. Stress, which may arise from worries, preoccupations, and troubling thoughts in the cerebral cortex, affects our bodies through the older health-regulating systems.

Likewise, researchers are accumulating evidence that depression, optimism, joy, and other emotional states may influence the immune or nervous systems in this way. But this communication is imperfect, because the older parts of the brain do not have language, a prime tool with which the cortex formulates messages. The practical outcome of this deficiency is that most of us cannot easily control the emotional, health-regulating parts of our brains through thoughts and ideas. We cannot easily regulate our blood pressure, control shivering, or alleviate fear simply by telling our brains and bodies to do so. At the same time, the healing portions of our brains may be reached in ways our rational thinking caps cannot easily comprehend. Trance, hypnosis, and other altered states of consciousness may bypass the cortex and reach directly into those deeper brain centers. Rituals, dance, drumming, and music may all soothe or stimulate us by appealing directly to those parts of the brain associated with emotion, regulation of the body, and healing.

Many mind-body therapies (discussed in Chapter Five) help people find more direct ways to control and communicate with the healing portions of their brains. Meditation and relaxation, for example, work by quieting the busily thinking cortex so the calming, healing brain centers can predominate. Imagery techniques also seek to reach older, deeper portions of the brain than those reached by words, thoughts, and ideas.

Many people find that through practice they can gain a measure of control over the areas of the brain that regulate bodily function—they can relax themselves, for example, or learn through biofeedback how to control mental states or motor nerves. Some people simply seem more skilled than others at such tasks. Among them may be those highly hypnotizable people discussed in Chapter One, who can translate mental images into burns on the skin. Some people seem better able to reach those portions of the brain that can effect bodily changes.

Is it possible that these abilities are part of a new trend in the evolution of the brain? We cannot know from our narrow perspective. But it is intriguing to wonder what direction evolution will take, whether brains in the distant future will have clearer communication between the thinking cap and the parts of the brain that control healing.

The discovery seemed to confirm what scientists had suspected—that the body makes its own morphinelike chemicals. Why else would the receptors exist? There would be no reason for the locks to have evolved if the body did not make keys to fit them. The search for internal pain-fighting drugs began, and by 1979 more than a half dozen *endorphins*—a contraction of the words *endogenous*, meaning "inside," and *morphine*—had been identified.

The discovery of endorphins and their receptors had profound implications for mind-body science. Not only were endorphins themselves mind-body chemicals—blocking pain and producing mild euphoria—but they suggested that there was a whole class of such chemicals. Structurally, endorphins are peptides, chains of amino acids. More specifically, they are called neuropeptides, because they are released from nerve endings. Scientists wondered if, in addition to the endorphins, there might not exist a system of neuropeptides active throughout the brain and body. Using new techniques, researchers looked for these minuscule messengers and found them flowing out of the hypothalamus and into the pituitary, the body's "master gland," which helps regulate dozens of bodily processes, including the release of flight-or-flight stress hormones from the adrenal glands. Neuropeptides, which frequently mimic the action of mood-altering drugs, were also found in other parts of the limbic system—that portion of the brain critical to drives and emotions. These findings led Pert and others to the startling conclusion that neuropeptides might be the "biochemicals of emotion." Each emotion, Pert reasoned, might be the result of a unique combination of neuropeptides. Pert—who spent twelve years at the National Institutes of Mental Health, where she advanced to chief of the brain biochemistry section before her departure in 1987—became deeply involved in the search for neuropeptides and their receptors. Because she found them, among other places, throughout the lining of the intestines, she proposed a new meaning for the old phrase gut feeling. Through the neuropeptide system, Pert reasoned, people might very well experience feelings in their guts.

If neuropeptides were linked to emotion, Pert

Only humans cry for purely emotional reasons, and the idea that crying can be healthy is a long-standing tradition in Western culture. More than two thousand years ago, Aristotle asserted that crying "cleanses the mind." And who has not heard the cliché "What you need is a good cry"? In one study, 85 percent of women and 73 percent of men reported that they felt better after crying. Research is beginning to suggest why we cry and how crying may promote not only emotional release but physical health.

One series of studies has focused on the biochemical composition of tears. At the Dry Eye and Tear Research Center at the St. Paul-Ramsey Medical Center in Minnesota, researcher William Frey showed subjects a tear-jerker movie and collected their tears in a small test tube. A few days later, the same subjects returned and were again prompted to weep, this time by being exposed to the aroma of a cut onion. Frey discovered that the emotional tears contained

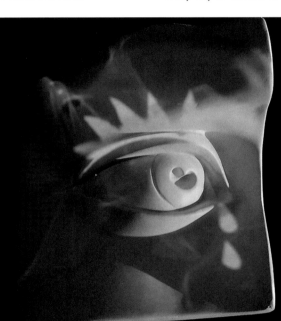

more protein than the tears released as a result of the eye irritant. He also discovered that both kinds contained bodily stress chemicals, specifically adrenocorticotropic hormone (ACTH), released by the pituitary gland, and leucine enkephalin, a morphinelike stress compound that may help mediate pain.

Another stress chemical in tears—called prolactin—may help explain why women cry four times more often than men. Prolactin is a hormone that helps stimulate the production of milk in women. Might women cry more often because they have naturally higher levels of this hormone? One bit of supportive evidence is that when prolactin levels drop after menopause, women sometimes suffer from dry-eye syndrome, in which the tear ducts do not produce enough tears. Drugs that retard prolactin production have also been found to produce dry-eye syndrome.

This research suggests that one reason we may cry is to lower the level of stress chemicals that can eventually erode health. According to this theory, the willingness to cry when under emotional pressure may help prevent stress-related disease.

Although scientists are far from proving this connection, a study at Marquette University has established a tentative link between attitudes toward crying and disease. Researchers interviewed one hundred men and women suffering from stress-related gastrointestinal disorders and compared their views on crying with those of healthy volunteers. Those suffering from the disorders were more likely than their healthy counterparts to view crying as a sign of emotional weakness. Continuing research may establish that emotional crying not only cleanses the mind but, as Aristotle believed, cleanses and heals the body as well.

wondered, could they also be linked to immunity and through immunity to the control of disease? Working with immunologist Michael Ruff, Pert began to study the effect of neuropeptides on monocytes, macrophages, and other immune cells. The researchers discovered neuropeptide receptors on all the primary cells of the immune system. In their studies of macrophages, every neuropeptide they tried—from opiate drugs to internal chemicals—altered the timing or direction of the cell's response.

Other researchers have shown not only that immune cells can listen to chemical messages, but that they can talk back in the same language. In a series of experiments that began in 1979, Dr. Ed Blalock of the University of Alabama found that white blood cells make many of the same hormones and neuropeptide messengers secreted by glands and nerve endings, and he suggested that through these chemicals the immune system can talk to every other system of the body. This ability to transmit, as well as receive, information has led some researchers to think of the immune system as a sensory organ for the rest of the body, constantly reporting on the status of immune cells, the presence of invaders, and other vital data. The resulting picture is of a new and radically different immune system. In the nearly forty years since the earliest experiments on stress and immune function, we have moved from the belief that the immune system acts independently of the brain, to the belief that the immune system may be influenced by the brain, to a new conception entirely: that the brain and the immune system may be part of an integrated system, working together for the body's health.

Science and the Healing System

Do any of these findings get us closer to answering the big question raised by Carl Simonton and others? Have we established that the mind-body links are clear enough to say that attitude or emotion can prompt the immune system to cure disease? The answer is both yes and no. Research has destroyed our belief that the mind plays no role in health. At the same time, we have learned how extraordinarily complicated the language of health and illness is. In a way, the more we learn, the less confident we are in

saying that any one variable promotes health or produces disease. Some researchers believe we are at the beginning of a new medical revolution more staggering than that of the nineteenth century. The emerging medical science is restoring the mind to the body. Health will increasingly be seen as both a physical state and a set of attitudes, both of which are irrevocably interdependent.

In his 1981 book, *Human Options*, American journalist Norman Cousins proposed a healing system activated by human belief and incorporating all of the body's resources that fight disease. If such a system exists, we are about as prepared to understand it as nineteenth-century scientists were to understand the immune system. We have seen the system at work—in the placebo response, in healing under hypnosis, in the extraordinary cures of spontaneous remission—but we have just begun to trace the mechanisms by which it works.

In theory, we should be able to study the healing system as we have studied the immune system and the body's other systems that control health. PNI is unveiling the mechanisms for one part of the system: those bodily components and processes that lend themselves to the methods of Western science. But we have only just begun to speculate on the other pathways: the ones between the body and the world outside. We have only the sketchiest idea of how a thought or feeling might be translated into electrical impulses in the brain or how they might find ultimate shape in the neuropeptide messengers Pert calls the "biochemicals of emotion." What we do know about these pathways tells us that they may work especially efficiently under meditation, trance, hypnosis, and other altered states of mind. The implication is that there may be ways of training people to enhance the efficiency of their healing pathways.

Ultimately, the mechanisms of healing may not be established under the rules of today's scientific medicine. During the revolution in medical science that is to come, the healing system may be understandable in a way that transcends current standards of proof, for that is what revolutions in thought are about: new ways of knowing and reinterpreting our position and purpose in the universe.

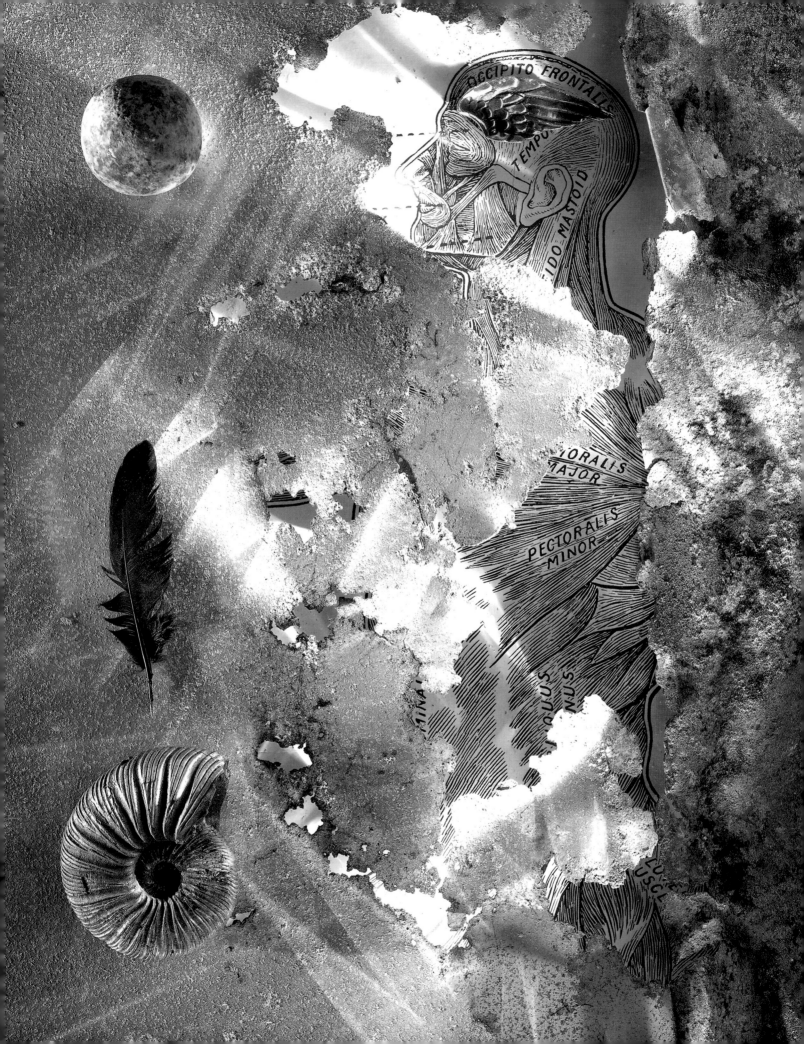

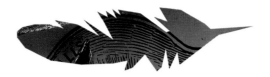

CHAPTER FOUR

WHO GETS SICK

PERSONALITY, EMOTION, AND HEALTH

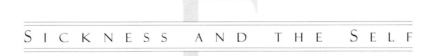

S I C K N E S S   A N D   T H E   S E L F

ACH YEAR THE U.S. ARMY selects about 7 percent of its most promising mid-level officers for advanced training. At the Army War College in Carlisle, Pennsylvania, some of these select men—and so far they mostly *are* men—enter a rigorous program of physical training and leadership-development classes. These officers are the army's elite: self-confident, hard-driving, assertive, persistent, eager to assume command, seeking perfection in themselves and others. But sometimes these qualities—so essential in leadership—manifest in other, less desirable traits. Dr. Meyer Friedman, a consultant for the army, uses the code AIAI to describe these traits—anger, impatience, arousal, and irritability. Friedman describes persons with Type A personalities as suffering from "hurry sickness": They are hostile and impatient, locked in perpetual struggle against one force or another—against time, against "the system," against their own high expectations for themselves and others. Friedman, a cardiologist, first became interested in Type A behavioral traits in the 1950s for the same reason the army did—because evidence indicates there might be a correlation between these traits and health. Not only are Type A officers more likely to die of heart disease, the

> *"It is better to know the patient that has the disease than the disease that has the patient."* —WILLIAM OSLER

army has found, but they also may make dangerous mistakes in judgment and put undue stress on those around them.

Today, every officer entering the War College is interviewed by a psychologist and, if necessary, placed in a stress-management workshop. "Do you walk fast?" the psychologist will ask an officer during the screening interview. "Do you eat fast?" "Do you like to do two or more things at the same time?" "Does your wife try to get you to slow down and take things easier?" "Do you feel your wife is too critical of you?" "In conversations with three or more people, do you believe these people speak to one another more than to you?" As important as the answers themselves are the officer's physical reactions and body language during the interview. An interviewer will look for signs of tension: lines between the eyes, a thickening of the jaw muscles from constant clenching, a muscle tic in the shoulders, and an angry, intent look around the eyes and mouth.

In the 1950s, when Dr. Friedman and his fellow cardiologist Dr. Raymond Rosenman coined the term "Type A behavior," medical science was just beginning to outline such risk factors for heart disease as cigarette smoking, a high blood-cholesterol level, genetic predisposition, lack of exercise, and a tendency to be overweight. Meanwhile, Friedman and Rosenman were becoming convinced that psychological factors also contributed to one's risk— that some people were at risk of heart disease simply because of the way they dealt with the world. One early clue came from a workman hired to reupholster the chairs in Friedman's outer office. According to Friedman's book, *Treating Type A Behavior and Your Heart*, the upholsterer wanted to know what kind of patients the doctor treated, and why the seats of the chairs were worn only on the front edge. Friedman didn't think much about the questions at the time, but later he began to wonder what tic of impatience his patients might have that would make them sit forward in their chairs.

Another clue emerged in 1956, during a study in

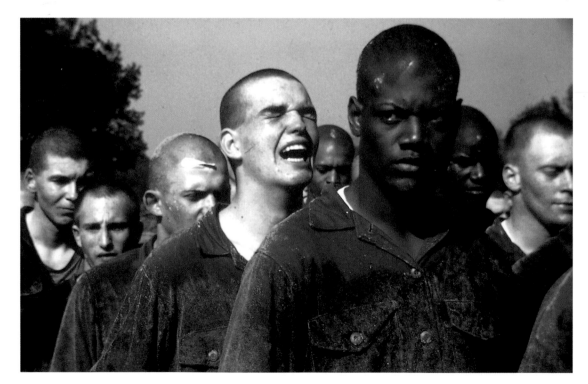

Hard-driving competitiveness, so useful in soldiering, can easily manifest in the Type A traits of anger, hostility, and impatience. Studies have shown that such traits put a person at great risk for heart diseases as do high blood pressure and high levels of blood cholesterol.

TEMPER TEST

A quick temper is among Type A traits sometimes associated with heart disease. Are you a hothead or relatively slow to anger? Take this test to find out.

A number of statements that people have used to describe themselves are given below. Read each statement and then circle the appropriate number to indicate how you generally feel. There are no right or wrong answers. Do not spend too much time on any one statement, but give the answer that seems to describe how you *generally* feel.

	Almost never	Sometimes	Often	Almost always
I am quick-tempered.	1	2	3	4
I have a fiery temper.	1	2	3	4
I am a hotheaded person.	1	2	3	4
I get angry when I'm slowed down by others' mistakes.	1	2	3	4
I feel annoyed when I am not given recognition for doing good work.	1	2	3	4
I fly off the handle.	1	2	3	4
When I get mad, I say nasty things.	1	2	3	4
It makes me furious when I am criticized in front of others.	1	2	3	4
When I get frustrated, I feel like hitting someone.	1	2	3	4
I feel infuriated when I do a good job and get a poor evaluation.	1	2	3	4

Score yourself: Counting the points (1 to 4) that you score on each item, add up the total and find where it places you in the percentile ranks. A man who scores 17, or a woman who scores 18, are just about average, at the 50th percentile. A person scoring below 13 is down in the safe zone, perhaps unresponsive to situations that provoke others. A score of 23 or higher puts you up among the hotter heads.

American Health, April 1983.

Percentile Ranks for Trait Anger

Percentile Ranks	Trait Anger	
	Females	Males
95	28	28
85	23	23
75	21	21
50	18	17
25	15	14
5	12	11

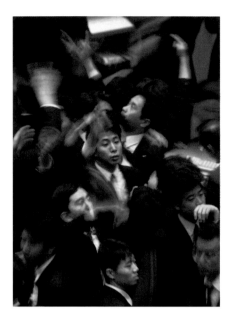

Jobs requiring unconditional attention and split-second decisions may contribute to health-eroding stress. These men are traders on the floor of the Tokyo stock exchange.

which Dr. Friedman and Dr. Rosenman closely recorded the diets of forty-six members of San Francisco's Junior League women's club and their husbands. The diets of the women were as high in animal fat and cholesterol as the men's, but the women were far less susceptible to heart disease. "If you really want to know what's going to give our husbands heart attacks, I'll tell you," the Junior League president told Friedman. "It's the stress they have to face in their businesses, day in, day out. Why, when my husband comes home at night, it takes at least one martini just to unclench his jaws."

One study neatly demonstrated how persistent stress might eventually lead to heart attack. Beginning in January 1957, researchers regularly drew blood from forty accountants to measure blood clotting and cholesterol levels, since fast clotting and high levels of cholesterol can cause clogged heart arteries and lead to heart attack. The study was planned to coincide with the income tax season, when many accountants struggle long hours to prepare clients' taxes. Sure enough, as the months passed, the accountants' blood clotted more easily and their cholesterol levels rose steadily, reaching a peak just before April 15, the most stressful day in any accountant's year. Following tax day, clotting times and cholesterol levels both returned to normal. (A similar effect has since been observed in officers at the Army War College, whose cholesterol levels remain steady during the eight-month course of study, except for a brief surge in January, the month the army announces which officers will be eligible for plum, fast-track assignments in the spring.)

In 1960, Dr. Friedman and Dr. Rosenman undertook a major study that would clearly establish the role of personality in at least one disease. The researchers divided 3,500 healthy men into two approximately equal groups—those who exhibited typical Type A behavior and those who did not. Eight and a half years later, they found that almost 70 percent of the men who had had heart attacks were in the Type A group. Type As were between two and three times more likely to suffer new heart attacks. The National Heart, Lung and Blood Institute carefully reviewed this study and concluded that not only was Type A behavior a risk factor in heart disease but it posed as great a danger as high blood pressure, high cholesterol levels, and smoking. Never had the role of attitude and behavior in a disease received such high-level endorsement.

What Makes People Sick?

The linking of Type A behavior to heart disease was a medical milestone. In the 1950s, "psychosomatic" diseases were still thought to be in a special class, somehow less "real" than "physical" ailments such as heart disease. The Type A research blurred the line between these classes of diseases. Although researchers had not yet established exactly *which* Type A traits were implicated in heart disease, it was now clear that even this manifestly physical disease was somehow linked to personality. The research also caught the imagination of the public and introduced the

Short self-tests, such as the ones below, may give some indication of a person's personality structure and the stresses encountered in everyday life. The tests below, for optimism (left) and pessimism (right), incorporate special scoring techniques to prevent "fooling" the tests. Take each test before you read about the scoring.

LIFE ORIENTATION TEST (LOT)

Please answer the following questions about yourself by indicating the extent of your agreement by using the following scale:

0—strongly disagree
1—disagree
2—neutral
3—agree
4—strongly agree

Be as honest as you can throughout, and try not to let your responses to one question influence your response to other questions. There are no right or wrong answers.

1. In uncertain times, I usually expect the best.
2. It's easy for me to relax.
3. If something can go wrong for me, it will.
4. I always look on the bright side of things.
5. I'm always optimistic about my future.
6. I enjoy my friends a lot.
7. It's important for me to keep busy.
8. I hardly ever expect things to go my way.
9. Things never work out the way I want them to.
10. I don't get upset too easily.
11. I'm a believer in the idea that "every cloud has a silver lining."
12. I rarely count on good things happening to me.

Score yourself:
1. Reverse code items 3, 8, 9, and 12. (On these items only, where you have scored 0, score 4, where you have scored 1, score 3, and vice versa. Scores of 2 remain unchanged.)
2. Sum items 1, 3, 4, 5, 8, 9, 11, and 12.
Note: Items 2, 6, 7, and 10 are filler items only. They are not scored as part of the scale. The maximum score on the test is 32. High scores indicate optimism; low scores reflect pessimism.

JOB STRESS INDEX: ARE YOU HASSLED?

This survey lists 10 job-related events that have been identified as stressful by employees working in different settings. Read each item and circle the number that indicates the approximate number of times during the past month that you have been upset or bothered by each event.

Number of occurrences during past month
(0, 1, 2, or 3+)

1. I have been bothered by fellow workers not doing their job.
2. I've had inadequate support from my supervisor.
3. I've had problems getting along with co-workers.
4. I've had trouble getting along with my supervisor.
5. I've felt pressed to make critical on-the-spot decisions.
6. I've been bothered by the fact that there aren't enough people to handle the job.
7. I've felt a lack of participation in policy decisions.
8. I've been concerned about my inadequate salary.
9. I've been troubled by a lack of recognition for good work.
10. I've been frustrated by excessive paperwork.

Score yourself: To determine how your stress compares with other workers, add up the points that you circled for each item (0–3). Your score will be between 0 and 30. Persons who score between 5 and 7 are about average in how often they experience job-related stress. If you score higher than 9, you may have cause for concern. At 4 or lower, you have a relatively non-stressful job.

American Health, April 1983.

Life Orientation Test, from *Health and Psychology*, vol. 4, 1985.
Reprinted with permission from Lawrence Erlbaum Associates, Inc.

EFFECTS OF BEHAVIORAL FACTORS ON IMMUNE MEASUREMENTS

Negative States and Traits

State/Trait	Reported Effects on Immune Measures
Bereavement	Decreased lymphocyte proliferation.
Pessimistic explanatory style	Decreased T-cell effectiveness; decreased lymphocyte reactivity
Academic/examination stress	Decreased NK cell activity; decreased T-cells; decrease in certain immune chemicals; increased susceptibility to herpes virus; decreased Immunoglobulin A; increased blood levels of Epstein-Barr virus.
Depression	Decreased number and function of lymphocytes; decreased NK cells; decreased T-cells.
Loneliness	Decreased NK activity.
Chronic stress	Decreased B-cells; decreased NK cells; decreased T-cells; increased blood levels of Epstein-Barr virus.
Divorce/separation/poor marital quality	Decreased lymphocyte function; increased blood levels of Epstein-Barr virus; decreased T-cell effectiveness.
Expressed need for power and control	Decreased NK activity; decreased lymphocytes.
Negative behavior during discussion of marital problems (high negative compared to low negative responses)	Decreased NK activity; decreased macrophages; increased blood levels of Epstein-Barr virus; increase in certain T-cells; decreased immunity by mitogen tests.

Positive States and Traits

Satisfying personal relationships and social support	Increased lymphocyte function; increased immunity by mitogen tests; increased NK activity; increased immune response to hepatits B vaccine.
Personal sharing and disclosure of traumatic experiences	Increased lymphocyte response.
Humor and laughter	Increased Immunoglobulin A; increased lymphocyte count and activity.
Hypnosis and relaxation techniques	Increased T-cell effectiveness; decreased blood levels of stress hormones; increased NK cell activity; decreased blood levels of herpes virus.
Physical exertion and aerobic exercise	Increased number of white blood cells; increase in endorphins; increase in certain immune chemicals; increased NK cell number and activity; increased T-cells; decreased T-cell effectiveness; decreased lymphocyte function.
Group intervention and support	Increased NK cell number and activity; increased number of lymphocytes; decrease in T-helper cells.

term Type A to the vocabulary of the street. Soon people were analyzing which of their friends had Type A personalities. At home, at the office, or at social gatherings, any flair of impatience or anger might elicit a quick admonition, "Don't be so Type A."

People are fascinated by the links between personality and disease. Creating categories is a central way humans make sense of the world, and it is only natural that we try to categorize people by common features and then link these features to human affliction. People have been attempting to make this connection since the beginning of written medical history. The humoral theory of disease, which dominated Western medical thinking for sixteen centuries, emphasized the links between personality and various ailments. Even after the growth of scientific medicine, with its focus on germs and mechanical causes of disease, some physicians continued to notice that certain sorts of people seemed to get certain diseases.

In 1910, for example, forty years before Meyer Friedman created the term Type A, pioneering physician William Osler offered a succinct characterization of the person at risk for heart disease. Such an individual was "robust," Osler wrote, "vigorous in mind and body, the ambitious man, the indicator of whose engines is always 'full speed ahead.' " By the 1970s, researchers were attempting to link specific personality traits and mental attitudes not only to heart disease but to headaches, cancer, stomach problems, allergy, rheumatoid arthritis, and mental breakdown. Although many of these studies have confirmed, in a general way, the age-old assumption that certain people suffer from certain ailments, they have also suggested that this link is not a simple one. Each person is a unique bundle of relatively stable *personality traits*, overlaid by more temporary emotional states and colored by ever-shifting moods and feelings. We have begun in the most rudimentary ways to associate specific traits with disease, but the uniqueness of human makeup and experience makes it difficult to generalize from one person to the next.

In studies of heart disease, for example, less attention is being focused on the global Type A personality and more on specific traits. General hurriedness and impatience now are viewed as less dangerous to the heart than hostility, barely controlled anger surging through the body. Some researchers believe that frequent waves of anger raise bodily stress chemicals, which in turn damage the heart and increase cholesterol levels. Research has shown that hostility alone can predict a person's susceptibility to heart disease and that certain other Type A traits may in fact promote health. More recently, hostility is being studied in its component parts—for example, suspiciousness, resentment, cynical mistrust, frequent anger—to see if any of these traits are more closely linked to heart disease.

Much emphasis in mind-body medicine has been placed on coping strategies, the way people deal with stress. But our reactions to stress depend not only on our personality but also on when the stress occurs

Opposite page: This chart summarizes data from more than twenty studies on the effects of various personal traits and states on immune function. Personality traits are often lifelong ways of approaching the world; states are more temporary. The data in such studies are based on statistical averages, so the correlations are certainly not hard and fast. The studies reflect, in a general way, how personality and personal experience may affect health.

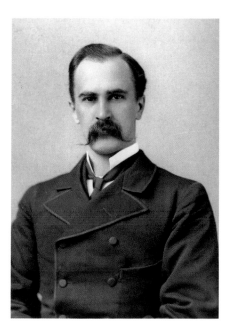

Dr. William Osler, shown here in 1881, was an influential Canadian physician associated with Johns Hopkins University Medical School and Oxford University.

Considered the most eminent clinician of his time, Osler stressed the role of emotion in illness and the importance of the patient's faith in recovery from disease.

and the other circumstances of our lives at the time. Researchers must also consider how personality and attitude may relate to other factors that affect health and our susceptibility to disease. The genes we inherit influence our health, as do a multitude of physical environmental factors, beginning in the womb and lasting throughout life. These include what we eat, the air we breath, how much exercise we get, and our exposures to microorganisms, carcinogens, and other poisons. To the extent that personality may influence health and disease, it always does so in interaction with these genetic and environmental factors—and perhaps with other influences we do not yet understand. With rare exceptions, no single factor—psychological or otherwise—is the simple cause of any disease.

Personality Precursors of Disease

Nonetheless, evidence is accumulating that psychological makeup can sometimes be as important as physical makeup in predicting who will get a certain illness and who will not. Most of this evidence has come from two kinds of studies: *retrospective* and *prospective*. In retrospective studies,

Psychologists often use a series of inkblots to identify personality traits and states. What a person sees in an inkblot may reflect unconscious tendencies and preoccupations. Psychologists work from keys telling them what most people see in each image, but uncommon responses are less important than the responses overall. The most famous test of this type is named for its creator, Hermann Rorshach, a Swiss psychiatrist who developed the test in 1911. This image comes from a different, but similar, test.

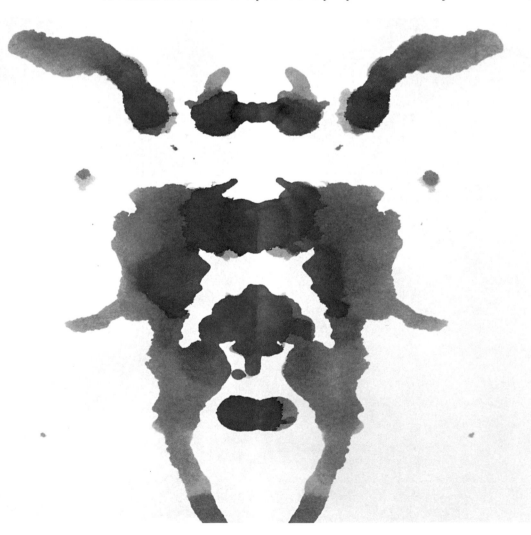

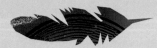

Since AIDS emerged as a recognized disease in the early 1980s, the news of its spread has been generally grim. The World Health Organization estimates that as of late 1992, two million people have developed AIDS worldwide and perhaps ten million more have been infected with the virus. According to the United States Centers for Disease Control and Prevention, 250,000 Americans had been diagnosed with AIDS by the end of September 1992. Of that number, 160,372 had died. But obscured by these statistics is at least a little heartening news: Some patients live far longer than expected, and a few patients who were diagnosed early in the epidemic are still alive today. In 1988, *Parade* magazine began following sixteen persons with AIDS who at that time had survived for more than three years since diagnosis. By early 1993, six of those people were still alive and leading active lives, including a few who had survived for more than ten years. Life for them was not only a precious gift but a genuine medical surprise.

Long-term survivors of AIDS and other deadly diseases offer dramatic anecdotal evidence that individual differences play a significant role in health, although no one knows what that role may be. Researchers have been naturally curious about the role of attitude and personality in these survivors. One researcher who has studied AIDS survivors is psychiatrist and PNI pioneer George Solomon, of the University of California, Los Angeles. Solomon became interested in patients with HIV infection and radically low T-cell counts who,

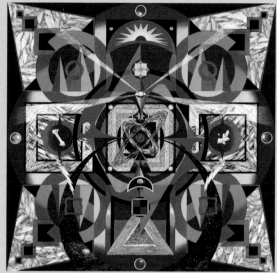

Artist King Thackston finds that mandalas, such as *The Serpent Wheels Begin to Turn* (above), "can work like healing meditations," and he uses them as centering devices.

for some reason, survive for long periods without AIDS symptoms. Solomon's studies involve small numbers of patients and the results are not statistically significant, but they suggest similarities in AIDS survivors:

• Many survivors have unfulfilled commitments in life and plans for the future. Ironically, many have discovered a new sense of meaning and purpose as a result of their illness. They see illness as a challenge rather than a threat. Many reach out to support other AIDS patients in hospice, home-care, and self-help groups. Others work to educate the public about HIV or lobby for funds for AIDS research.

• In caring for their own health, most survivors react with neither compliance nor defiance to their doctors' suggestions, but see themselves as educated partners in their own care. They assume personal responsibility for that care and in doing so achieve a sense of self-efficacy, a sense that what they do affects how they feel and how their disease progresses.

• Most survivors enjoy social support, people they can talk to about their fears and concerns. At the same time, they have developed a sensitivity to their own physical and psychological needs, an ability to withdraw from outside commitments and take care of themselves when necessary. In one study of AIDS patients, the ability to say "no" to a requested favor correlated highest with improved immunity.

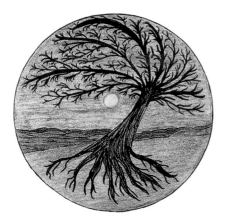

"The roots represent tumors, and the need to hold on — to plant myself firmly in the ground, instead of leaving. They reflect the feelings going on within me." The paintings on these two pages were created by Laurie Downs, a cancer patient, during the three years she was part of an art therapy group eight years ago.

The circle enclosing each drawing is called a mandala, an art therapy technique taught her by Elizabeth Weathersby, a registered art therapist. Downs, who lives in Atlanta and has been in remission for five years, painted every day while she was sick, and still paints today.

a person is interviewed *after* getting sick in an effort to establish long-term personality characteristics. But since illness itself can affect personality, the most convincing studies are prospective, in which people are interviewed and then followed for years to see what illnesses they develop.

One of the most ambitious prospective studies was started in 1946 at Johns Hopkins University Hospital in Baltimore. Dr. Caroline Thomas wanted to study whether heart disease and high blood pressure could be predicted by physical exams and psychological tests given years in advance. If disease could be predicted, Dr. Thomas believed, perhaps a way could be found to prevent it. Because the study was looking for precursors of disease, it was called the Precursors Study. It is the longest-running such study in American medical history.

Thomas found the subjects for her study close at hand. Between 1946 and 1964, all Johns Hopkins medical students—more than 1,330 of them—received a battery of questionnaires, physical examinations, and psychological tests. Among the questionnaires was one that assessed typical reactions to nervous tension and stress. Another addressed the student's attitudes toward his parents and his perception of their attitudes toward him. Psychological tests included the Rorschach test, during which students described what they saw in a series of ambiguous inkblots, and a test in which each student drew a simple human figure. Decades later, all but a handful of these students, most of whom are doctors now, continue to send in health data several times each year.

If Dr. Thomas had thought that heart disease would claim the first of her former students, she was wrong. Much to her surprise, thirteen were already dead of suicide by the time the first subject suffered a heart attack, in 1965. Thomas and her colleagues went to the data from the examinations and questionnaires to see if these suicides could have been predicted—the answer was a tentative yes. The students who eventually committed suicide had reported irritability, the urge to be alone, frequent urination, difficulty sleeping, and the loss of appetite two to three times more often than the other subjects. During the inkblot test they were forty-six times more likely to use the phrase *crying for help*, twenty-four times more likely to use the word *drowning*, and fourteen times more likely to use the words *cancer* or *tumor* in describing an inkblot. More than five years before committing suicide, one man reported that the inkblot showed a "man with hand upraised, crying for help, drowning."

In 1973, a quarter century after the study was begun, Thomas and her fellow researchers reviewed the five major causes of death and disability among the former students—suicide, mental illness, hypertension, cancerous tumors, and coronary heart disease leading to heart attack. As expected, the researchers found significant biological precursors to many of these conditions. Subjects suffering from high blood pressure, for example, had recorded the highest blood pressures as students and had been more likely to be overweight. Those who had suffered heart attacks

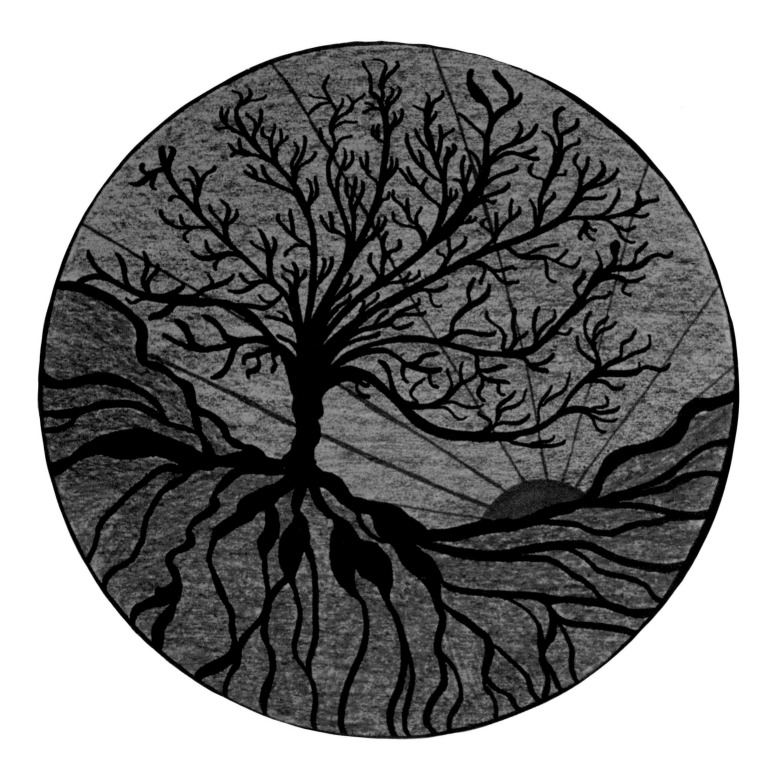

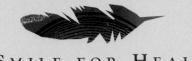

Most of us understand instinctively that emotions have physical components. For example, fear can provoke a stress response, in which the heart and breathing quicken and blood is shunted to the large muscles to prepare for fight or flight. Likewise, anger, happiness, sadness, disgust, and surprise each prompts physical responses that make us "feel" a particular way. These responses form one likely link between emotions and health. But how much control do we have over our emotional states? Are emotions simply reactions, or can we force ourselves to be happy or sad? Does it do any good to follow the advice of the old song and simply "put on a happy face"? According to University of California psychologists Paul Ekman and Robert Levenson, following this advice may actually make us feel better when we're low. Ekman, who has been interested in smiles, frowns, grimaces, glowers, and grins for decades, has discovered that facial expressions are universal across cultures and are linked neurologically to emotional states.

Ekman and Levenson have demonstrated that facial expressions not only are reactions to emotional states but can provoke these states as well. In their experiments, the researchers directed subjects to move specific muscles in their face, but did not tell them what emotion the expression was supposed to connote. For example, subjects were directed to pull their eyebrows down and together, to raise their upper eyelids, and to push their lower lip up and press the lips together—forming a facial expression that connotes anger in every human culture. At the same time, the researchers measured four physiological variables that change with emotional states: heart rate, finger temperature, skin conductance, and muscle activity.

They also asked the subjects what feelings, sensations, or memories they experienced during each facial expression. Results showed that each emotional state is associated with physiological changes and that these changes can be reproduced through facial expression alone. In a significant number of instances, subjects also reported feelings that matched the facial expression they were asked to produce. In these subjects, looking angry not only made them feel angry but also caused their bodies to react as if they were angry.

Does this mean that someday depressed patients will be scheduled for smile therapy? Certainly it confirms the long-standing wisdom that if you're feeling down, forcing yourself to try to have a little fun will help you feel better. "Putting on a polite expression, going to a social gathering in which one has to smile and be polite may actually change how one feels," Ekman has written. The face we turn to the world may not only reflect our inner state but continually plays a role in shaping that experience as well.

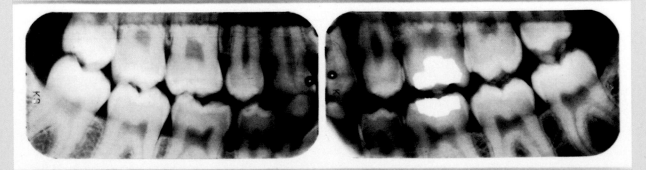

had smoked the most cigarettes as students and had shown the highest levels of blood cholesterol. Psychosocial factors were also associated with specific diseases and death—and not just among the suicides. Those who had been treated for heart disease had earlier been rated as closest to their parents of all of the illness groups. By contrast, those students who eventually got cancer had reported having the most distant relationships with their parents.

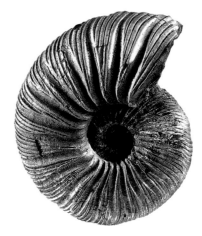

Cancer: The Nicest Patients

A distant relationship with one's parents was not the only psychosocial correlate of cancer in the decades-long Precursors Study. Subjects who would eventually develop cancer had reported the fewest habits of nervous tension as students and had received the lowest scores for depression, anxiety, and anger. A special analysis of their Rorschach responses showed them to be more likely than those of other students to reveal unsatisfactory relationships with others.

With the recent exception of AIDS, perhaps no disease fascinates and frightens us more than cancer. Although many cancers are now curable, the disease is associated in our imaginations with pain, disfigurement, and death. Cancer is second only to heart disease in the number of persons it kills in the United States each year. It is no accident that cancer and heart disease are the two diseases for which researchers most commonly claim a personality component. Both are complex, degenerative diseases that develop over a long time and become more common with age— exactly the kinds of diseases that might be correlated with long-term personality traits and attitudes. Cancer and heart disease are also among the most difficult diseases to cure; people suffering from the leading kinds of cancer are no more likely to survive today than they were a generation ago, and the incidence of several varieties of cancer is on the rise.

Cancer is a complicated disease in part because it is so various and so difficult to tie to any single cause. In a healthy person, body cells constantly reproduce in accordance with internal control; in a cancer patient, this control somehow breaks down, causing cells to multiply chaotically. This process might be facilitated by an inherited weakness or by damage to the body by environmental carcinogens. In addition, a multitude of conditions may weaken the immune system's ability to detect and eliminate abnormal cells, allowing a cancer to take hold and grows. Some researchers suggest that, by diminishing a person's immune response, psychological factors may tip the scale toward the development of certain types of cancer.

Many scientists believe that cancer is primarily a biological process in which psychological and social factors play a minor and yet undetermined role. Other researchers and some patients, however, believe that the link between personality and cancer can be significant. Alice Epstein, for example, was a sixty-five-year-old Massachusetts woman in 1985 when her doctors gave her three months to live. Epstein's

> *"This is a success story based on love and the willingness to go deeply into yourself, and to move from confusion into happiness."*
>
> —ALICE EPSTEIN

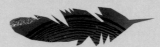

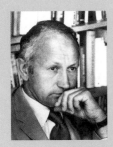

In 1976, American journalist Norman Cousins announced that he had cured himself of a serious illness partly through hearty belly laughs. Cousins had been stricken with alkylosing spondylitis, an often fatal degenerative disease of the spine. His worried doctor quickly hospitalized Cousins and put him on four different medications to relieve his pain and inflammation, but the doctor held little hope that Cousins would ever recover. But Cousins had been a medical writer before becoming editor of *Saturday Review* magazine. He was aware of emerging evidence that depression and pessimism can decrease resistance to disease and produce negative effects on the body. If bad feelings could harm the body, Cousins reasoned, might not good feelings produce positive results?

With the close cooperation of his doctor, Cousins became a take-charge participant in his own care. He stopped taking most of his medicines, and convinced his doctor to order massive doses of vitamin C, which Cousins believed might help combat the inflammation. But the centerpiece of his treatment was a deliberate courting of positive emotions. "It was easy enough to hope and love and have faith," Cousins wrote in *Anatomy of an Illness*, his best-selling book about the experience, "but what about laughter? Nothing is less funny than being flat on your back with all the bones in your spine and joints hurting."

Cousins requested a movie projector and screen for his room and watched old Marx Brothers films and episodes of the TV series "Candid Camera." He also had nurses read to him from humorous books. "I made the discovery that ten minutes of genuine belly laughter had an anesthetic effect and would give me at least two hours of pain-free sleep," Cousins reported. Out of curiosity, Cousins's doctor began sampling his blood sedimentation rate—a crucial measure of inflammation—before and after each laugh session. The sedimentation rate fell slightly with each session, and continued to fall as Cousins gradually recovered.

In 1976, when Cousins first published an account of his case in the *New England Journal of Medicine*, there was little scientific evidence to support the age-old biblical notion that "a merry heart doeth good like a medicine." Since then, studies have found not only that laughter reduces stress and eases pain, but that it seems to alter the basic body chemistry of stress and immunity. For one study, blood samples were drawn from ten healthy subjects at ten-minute intervals and tested for eight different hormones and biochemical messengers. Half the experimental group simply sat quietly for an hour as the blood was drawn. The other half watched a sixty-minute videotape of a performance of the comedian Gallagher. Members of that group showed a significant decrease in cortisol and epinephrine, two stress hormones that are known to decrease immune function.

Other studies have shown that laughter spurs the production of antibodies in the upper respiratory track and increases the action of lymphocytes and the all-important natural killer cells, which are particularly active against viruses and tumors. And we have long known that laughter is good exercise—expanding the lungs, increasing heart rate, and stimulating the muscles.

Based on such studies and on years of observation that happy patients seem to heal faster, hospitals around the country are launching programs to encourage laughter and other pleasant emotions. Some hospitals have created special activity rooms where patients go to watch a movie or listen to a favorite piece of music. In other hospitals, one channel of the patients' television network carries nonstop comedies, and special "laughter wagons" bring

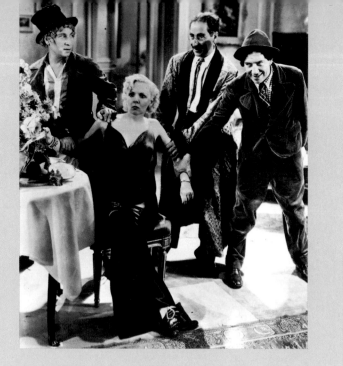

Opposite page:
Norman Cousins.
Above: A scene
from the Marx
Brothers' movie, *A
Day at the Races.*

amusing books or gifts to the patients' bedsides. In one hospital, nurses were seen wearing buttons that read, "Warning: Humor may be hazardous to your illness."

Increasingly, other authorities are recognizing the healing power of laughter. In the last few years, for instance, psychologists and "laughter therapists" have offered workshops and retreats at which they teach corporate executives and others how to "lighten up" and enjoy a good laugh. It is a trend Cousins would endorse; he remained convinced of the power of belief and positive emotion in medicine throughout the rest of his life.

After retiring from journalism, Cousins was invited to become an adjunct professor at the University of California School of Medicine, where he taught young doctors about the importance of belief, faith, control, and positive emotions in healing. In 1980, Cousins suffered a massive heart attack, but he was soon back on the tennis court, convinced that "being caught up in pleasant activity had a great deal to do with cardiac capacity." His recovery from the heart attack was just one more example, he wrote, of "the importance of the will to live." Cousins died in 1990 at the age of seventy-eight.

energy had been flagging for months, and she was no longer able to keep up with her husband, Sy, when they went cross-country skiing in the woods near their home. She began taking long afternoon naps, and one day she was struck with excruciating pain. The diagnosis was kidney cancer that had spread to her lungs. Surgeons removed the cancerous kidney but could offer no treatment for the lesions in her lung, which were spreading rapidly and showed up as distinct spots on her chest x-ray. "I was distressed," Epstein said, "but not surprised."

She was not surprised because she believed she had the traditional cancer-prone personality. During the last four decades, researchers have sketched remarkably similar personality profiles for some people who either already have or will eventually acquire cancer. Epstein had taken personality tests and understood that she fit the pattern. Unlike Type A persons susceptible to heart attack, who lash out with anger and hostility at the least provocation, persons susceptible to cancer are thought to express anger only rarely. They are often the rock-solid support of their families, and ask for little support for themselves. Once diagnosed, these patients seem to accept their illness with remarkable calm and worry less about themselves than the suffering and inconvenience their cancer may cause others. Doctors describe them as "the nicest patients"—understanding, compliant, stoic, and uncomplaining.

How might such "Type C" behavior help promote cancer? Theorists speculate that when anger and other emotions are not expressed, they produce changes in the body's hormonal and mind-body control systems that may weaken immunity and allow a tumor to develop. "I was very aware of a connection between the way I had felt before I became ill and my illness," Epstein said. "I was unhappy. I knew that life was not the way it used to be." She described her personality as "always looking out for somebody else, and never looking out for myself."

Epstein's husband, Sy, a psychologist, soon became convinced there was a psychological dimension to his wife's disease. Sy remembers a walk he took with her soon after her diagnosis. It had begun to snow, and she had always loved the snow. She turned to him with tears in her eyes: "I'll never see another

THE HEART OF HEALING 101

HOLMES-RAHE SOCIAL READJUSTMENT SCALE

This scale was developed by physicians Richard Rahe and Thomas Holmes to reflect the disruptive effects of certain changes in a person's life. Dr. Holmes and Dr. Rahe suggested that a score exceeding 300 in one year indicated an 80 percent probability of developing serious illness. Because everyone reacts to change differently, the scale is best used as a general measure of the relative stress from life events.

Dr. Hans Selye first popularized the term "stresssed out" in the 1930s.

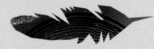

Rank	Life event	Mean value
1	Death of spouse	100
2	Divorce	73
3	Marital separation	65
4	Jail term	63
5	Death of close family member	63
6	Personal injury or illness	53
7	Marriage	50
8	Fired at work	47
9	Marital reconciliation	45
10	Retirement	45
11	Change in health of family member	44
12	Pregnancy	40
13	Sex difficulties	39
14	Gain of a new family member	39
15	Business readjustment	39
16	Change in financial state	38
17	Death of close friend	37
18	Change to different line of work	36
19	Change in number of arguments with spouse	35
20	Mortgage over $10,000	31
21	Foreclosure of mortgage or loan	30
22	Change in responsibilities at work	29
23	Son or daughter leaving home	29
24	Trouble with in-laws	29
25	Outstanding personal achievement	28
26	Wife begin, or stop, work	26
27	Begin or end school	26
28	Change in living conditions	28
29	Revision of personal habits	24
30	Trouble with boss	23
31	Change in work hours or conditions	20
32	Change in residence	20
33	Change in schools	20
34	Change in recreation	19
35	Change in church activities	19
36	Change in social activities	18
37	Mortgage or loan less than $10,000	17
38	Change in sleeping habits	16
39	Change in number of family get-togethers	15
40	Change in eating habits	15
41	Vacation	13
42	Christmas	12
43	Minor violation of the law	11

snowfall." "Suddenly this feeling of anger came over her," Sy remembered, "and she said 'I'm not going to die. I'm going to fight it with everything I have.' I was shocked with the intensity of it, and I also was delighted. And I said, 'I'll do everything I can to help you.' "

Epstein began an intensive program of psychotherapy and meditation. She found she was particularly skilled at exploring and expressing her feelings and emotions through fantasy. In daily therapy sessions, she began to visualize her emotions. She fantasized separate personalities for her feelings of aggressiveness, for her helplessness, for her ineffectual side. Within a few weeks, she could feel herself changing. After several months of meditation and psychotherapy, Epstein was approved for an experimental medical treatment—a last attempt to prolong her life. But before putting the needle in her arm, her doctor ordered a chest x-ray. The x-ray showed that the tumors in her lungs were shrinking, and Epstein decided against the experimental treatment. Within a year the tumors would completely disappear.

Technically, Epstein had experienced remission from lung metastases of kidney cancer after removal of the cancerous kidney. Although lung metastases from kidney cancer are the most likely of all cancers to remit spontaneously, such remissions are very rare. Why Epstein was one of these fortunate patients— and to what degree her psychological state was involved in her remission—we do not know for certain.

Epstein, however, has no doubts. "This illness forced me to deal with my personality," she said. "It forced me to be a different person. I don't say I enjoyed having cancer, but it was one of the best things that happened to me, because I'm now a different person. This is a success story based on love and the willingness to go deeply into yourself, and to move from confusion into happiness."

WHAT PEOPLE NEED FOR HEALTH

In the mid-1970s, a graduate student in psychology at the University of Chicago experienced a revelation while sitting in a doctor's waiting room. Suzanne Kobasa was paging through a magazine when she came across an article on stress, which included a do-it-yourself questionnaire based on a commonly used numerical scale of stressful life events. The scale had been developed about ten years earlier by physicians Richard Rahe and Thomas Holmes as a way of answering the question "Why do some people get sick while others don't?" The team interviewed thousands of people, asking them to rank the various stresses in their lives.

Based on the subjects' responses, the researchers assigned a stress rating to forty-three common life events: the death of a spouse carried the highest stress rating, of 100, and a minor violation of the law rated 11. The Holmes-Rahe Social Readjustment Scale (page 102) offered an objective measure for researchers trying to assess the effects of stress on health. It also recognized that not only negative or painful events were stressful—that any change could create stress, including marriage (stress rating 50) and an outstanding personal achievement (stress rating 28).

The researchers suggested that the higher a person's score rose above 300 points, the more likely the person was to develop a serious illness. But as Kobasa worked out her own score while sitting in her doctor's outer office, she found that her total easily topped 300. Not only was Kobasa not ill, but she felt in little danger of becoming so. Surely, she thought, the relationship between stress and disease must be more complicated than the Holmes-Rahe scale suggested. For example, the test did not account for the specific circumstances surrounding life events—a drawback Holmes and Rahe recognized. The death of a husband might carry a different degree of stress if he was a wife-beater than if he was a lifelong, beloved companion. An enormous church wedding, requiring months of preparation, might be more stressful than a quiet marriage ceremony. Kobasa took this argument even further: Might not identical life changes affect different people in different ways, depending on

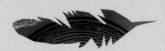

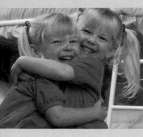

Mind-body research is confirming the age-old notion that health and personality may be related. But personality is, to various degrees, both inherited and shaped by later experience and is difficult to separate from other influences on health—from the genetic makeup we inherit from our parents, for example, to the environment in which we are raised. Some of the most helpful evidence in discerning these influences comes from studies of identical twins who were separated at birth and raised in different homes. Because such twins share almost exactly the same genetic makeup, they offer a rare opportunity to study what scientists call "the nature-nurture question."

Since 1979, scientists at the University of Minnesota have been studying adult twins raised in separate homes—many of whom did not even know of their twin's existence until the study brought them together. Each pair of twins in the study completes a six-day testing marathon. They are examined by psychologists, geneticists, dentists, and four varieties of physician. They are x-rayed, videotaped, wired to electrodes, and asked to answer fifteen thousand written questions on everything from their sexual history to their performance in school.

The results have revealed striking similarities. For example, twins from Ohio were separated in infancy but coincidentally given the same name—Jim—by their adoptive parents, worked for many years at the same job, drove the same kind of car, smoked the same brand of cigarette, and pursued the same hobby, woodworking. Both nervously bit their fingernails, and had developed migraines at the same age. Twins Jerry Levey and Mark Newman were both firefighters—for different communities in New Jersey—although neither twin knew of the other's existence until a friend of Mark spotted Jerry at a convention and brought the two men together. The resemblance was remarkable: the men sported identical

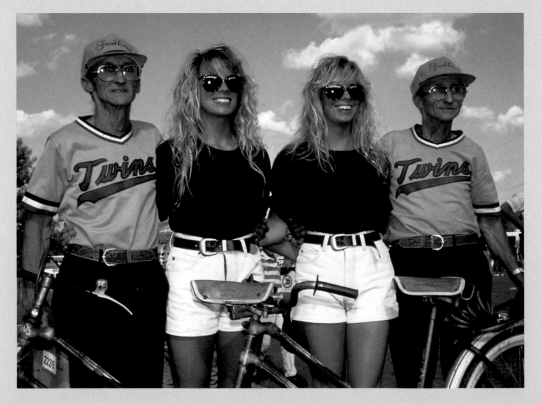

Identical twins—especially those separated at birth and raised in different homes—offer scientists a rare opportunity to study the relationship among personality, genetics, and health. This photo was taken at the annual Twins Days Festival in Twinsburg, Ohio.

bushy mustaches and sideburns and wore the same style eyeglasses. Both were good-humored bachelors and habitual flirts who drank only Budweiser.

The Minnesota study also suggests that encoded in our genes are predispositions to health and certain diseases. Identical twins in the study shared almost identical susceptibility to heart and lung diseases. Some twins had suffered from the same diseases at approximately the same point in life, including heart disease, diabetes, and pancreatitis. In one pair of identical triplets, researchers discovered the same rare eye disease. The study also suggests that a person is more likely to suffer from some mental disorders, including schizophrenia, anxiety, and phobias, if the person's twin has the disorder. Even the immune systems of identical twins are markedly similar.

Researchers emphasize that often it is not diseases that are inherited, but predispositions to diseases, and that these can be profoundly influenced by environment. A twin who smokes a pack of cigarettes each day is at greater risk of contracting lung cancer than a twin who does not smoke, no matter what their predisposition to the disease might be. In an effort to learn more about the inheritability of attitudes, emotional tendencies, and personality traits, which may themselves influence health, the researchers measured nearly a dozen personality traits, including traditionalism, need for achievement, social closeness, and sense of well-being. They concluded that about 50 percent of an individual's personality is a result of genetic predisposition, while the other 50 percent is shaped by family upbringing and a person's unique experiences. Such studies serve as a warning against making broad pronouncements about the link between personality and health, since both our psychological attributes and predisposition to disease seem to be intricately entwined with our genes.

personality? Might not some people be prepared to deal better with the stress because of their attitude toward themselves and the world?

This makes sense—it is not the stressful event itself that promotes health or illness, but our attitude toward that event. Few people would want to avoid the stress associated with a job promotion, an upcoming marriage, or the eagerly anticipated birth of a child. Such changes are also challenges and the very stuff that gives life meaning.

In her own research, Kobasa—now of the City University of New York— has tried to sort out exactly what personality traits help some people resist health-eroding stress. With colleague Salvatore Maddi, she began a study of middle- and upper-level employees of Illinois Bell, a large telephone company that was experiencing tremendous upheavals. The researchers wondered what personality characteristics would help these executives maintain health in the face of professional upheavals and through everyday changes in their personal lives.

Hardiness and Health

As the research progressed, three attitudes seemed to separate the executives labeled hardy by the researchers from the executives more likely to fall ill under stress. These attitudes—the "three Cs" of the hardy individuals—were commitment, control, and challenge. The hardy executives stayed committed and involved in whatever they were doing and in the experiences presented by life. This commitment, in turn, offered them a sense of purpose that gave meaning to their lives and environment. They eagerly undertook their work and obligations and were unlikely to give up under pressure. A sense of control gave the hardy executives a feeling of mastery over their circumstances; they were less likely to feel helpless in the face of change and more likely to perceive options in the face of stress. Finally, they were more likely to experience change as challenge rather than threat—as the norm rather than the exception—and therefore as less stressful. Decades of research have suggested the importance of such attitudes in the preservation of mental and physical health. People who believe they are in control of events, who are committed to their work and other

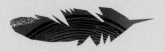

A young couple discusses problems in their six-month marriage. She thinks he could do the housework a little more often. He is worried that she is spending more money than they can afford. Sex is also a concern: she is often asleep when he comes to bed. "I know I always try to put you off, " she says. The setting is not the couple's apartment, but a hospital room in the clinical research center at Ohio State University. And although the issues are personal, the discussion is by no means taking place in private. The husband and wife sit facing one another, and a video camera is trained on each face, recording every nuance of expression. Each of them has a blood pressure cuff wrapped around one arm. The other arm is fitted with a catheter (for drawing blood) and pushed through an opening in a curtain beside their chairs. Behind the curtain, two nurses scan a bank of electronic monitors and periodically draw blood from the couple's arms. Like ninety other

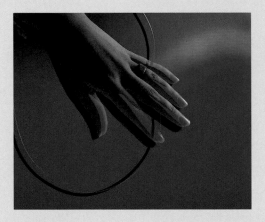

newlywed couples studied by Ronald Glaser and Janice Kiecolt-Glaser, this couple will stay in the research center for twenty-four hours and for much of that time will discuss their marital problems and pleasures. To study the effects of these interactions over time, nurses will draw blood from them even while they sleep.

The Glasers' study is but a small part of a gradually amassing body of material on the effects of marriage on immunity and health. Researchers have noted that social support and close relationships seem important to health, and in studying marriage, they are studying the closest relationship most adults ever develop. One of the findings of this research is that simply being married is not enough to maintain immunity. The Glasers and their associates compared the immune systems of thirty-eight

married women with those of thirty-eight women who had recently been separated or divorced. Marital disruption was found to decrease immunity, but so was the stress of living in a bad marriage.

One of the goals of the Glasers' research is to find out how marital interactions affect stress, stress chemicals, and immunity. On the one hand, they are discovering that pleasant interactions do not seem to affect physiology— they do not "boost" the immune system. On the other hand, some negative interactions clearly take a toll, especially on women, whose immune systems seem more sensitive to marital stress.

In both men and women, what seems to affect the immune system most is not *that* marital partners disagree but *how* they disagree. Interactions characterized by hostility, sarcasm, and blame—by refusing to take responsibility and demeaning the other partner—seem to be most damaging. Participants in such interactions show an increase in stress chemicals and a decrease in immunity that is still evident when the couple leaves the research center the next day. The researchers emphasize that such small immune changes in generally healthy and contented young people will probably not have much effect on their health. But what about long-term acrimonious relationships, in which the blaming and hostility go on for years? The Glasers plan to follow their newlyweds to discover if an ongoing bad relationship leads to long-term immune changes and greater susceptibility to disease.

"The quality of a relationship matters," said Kiecolt-Glaser, "especially for women. What our study is showing is that the physiological effects of marriage may be much stronger than we ever thought."

life goals, and who are invigorated and challenged by change are less likely to be knocked off course by the bumps and curves along life's road. Such persons also tend to be optimistic, to see more good in life than bad, to feel hope more often than helplessness.

Researchers have explored the role of control particularly, since it is relatively easy to study in laboratory animals. Experiments with rats and mice have shown that tumors grow faster in stressed animals than in unstressed animals. But when animals gain some measure of control over the stress—for example, when they can avoid being shocked by pressing a bar—tumor growth slows.

In several studies, rats experiencing controllable stress actually showed slower tumor growth or more tumor rejection than rats that were not stressed at all. For a study published in the journal *Science* in 1982, Madelon Visintainer implanted tumor cells in rats and then divided the rats into three groups. Visintainer already knew how many cells to implant so that under normal conditions about half the rats would reject the tumors. In her unstressed control group, that is exactly what happened—within a month, 50 percent of the rats rejected the tumors and the other 50 percent died. The second group of rats experienced regular shocks they could not control, and only 27 percent of those rats rejected their tumors. But of the third group of rats, which experienced shock that could be turned off by pressing a bar, 70 percent rejected the tumors. Being in control of the stress somehow seemed to increase the ability of the rats' immune systems to reject the tumors at a rate higher than normally would have been expected.

In our culture, many elderly people lose their sense of control over their lives. Experiments have shown that the elderly stay healthier and live longer, however, if they can maintain a measure of control. For a study published in 1976, researchers at Yale University divided nursing home residents into two groups, which were matched for disability and ill health. Both groups were offered amenities above the standard nursing home fare: special meals and entertainment, along with a plant for the bedside. One group was offered control over these extras; the other was not.

Each evening, the group A patients were asked to choose omelets or scrambled eggs for the next morning's breakfast. These patients were also required to sign up to attend special movie nights and had to choose their own bedside plants and see that they were cared for. The group B patients, by contrast, breakfasted on omelets or scrambled eggs on an unvarying schedule and were told which nights they would go to the movies. Nurses chose the plants for the group B patients and assumed all responsibility for the plants' care and watering. After only three weeks, the group A patients showed evidence of noticeably improved health, and after eighteen months only half as many of these patients had died as in group B.

The Importance of Optimism

Control, commitment, challenge, and a sense of purpose help prevent a sense of helplessness, hopelessness, and disabling depression. No mental attitude seems to bode as ill for health as the sense that all is lost. Many depressed people simply stop taking care of themselves and see little reason to get enough sleep, eat a healthful diet, drink alcohol in moderation, or avoid cigarette smoking or other dangerous habits. Hopelessness may also directly affect the body. When faced with unavoidable stress in experiments, many rats will die. The "voodoo death" witnessed in some human cultures may be caused by the same sense of hopelessness—that the curse is inevitable, beyond control. (See "Scared to Death," Chapter One.)

Hopelessness and depression have been associated with cancer since the second century, when the Greek physician Galen suggested that "melancholy" women seemed more susceptible to the disease. For one study of cancer and depression, researchers reviewed the death certificates of more than two thousand men and compared them with personality tests of the men given seventeen years before. Highly depressed men were more than twice as likely as other subjects to die from cancer.

Health-eroding feelings of helplessness, pessimism, and depression can be deeply imbedded in personality. Two people faced with exactly the same situation can react in almost opposite ways: one person may see a glass as half empty, and the other may see it as half

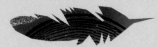

Humans are social animals—we seek out others of our species and join together to meet common goals. Without companionship, we may experience loneliness and separation, which are among the most painful human conditions. But why should connectedness be so central to the human experience? Many researchers believe the answer lies in the development of the fetus and the evolution of the human brain over millions of years, beginning when the ancestors of today's humans first descended from the trees to live on the plains of Africa.

Over the following millennia, our ancestors evolved a large brain that enabled them to adapt to a wide variety of environments, and, at the same time, they evolved a narrower, heavier pelvis to support the extra weight of standing erect. This presented an evolutionary problem: Larger brains require larger heads, but a baby with a large head is not easily born through a narrow pelvis. Over hundreds of thousands of years, an evolutionary compromise developed—human infants are genetically programmed to develop big brains, but their brains develop substantially after birth. The brain of the human newborn weighs only 25 percent of its adult weight, compared with the brain of a baboon newborn, whose brain weighs 70 percent of an adult's.

Few animals are born as helpless as the human being, and no creature stays so helpless for so long, so dependent on the ministrations of others. A newborn human requires at least one full-time caretaker for several years after birth—in most cultures, this is the baby's mother. In the hunter-gatherer culture of early humans, a young mother would have needed help to feed her very young dependent children and herself. Many anthropologists believe this is why the human family evolved: to feed and nurture the long-helpless young. This may be one reason many of us find separation from others so painful. The root of our connectedness and need for one another may be buried deep in the evolutionary wisdom of our species. No matter how sophisticated our culture becomes, there may be a part of us that continues to believe that if we are abandoned by others we will die.

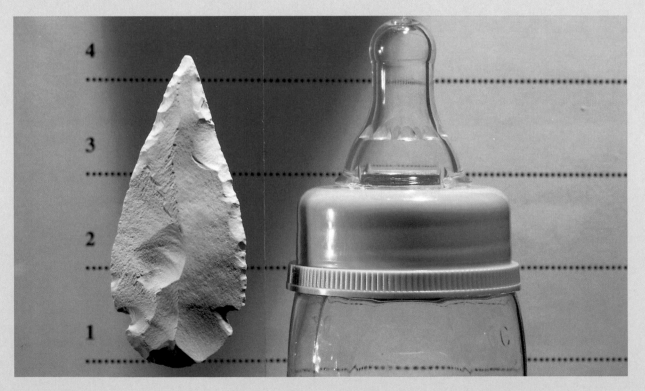

full. Psychologist Martin Seligman has dedicated his career to exploring how people learn optimistic or pessimistic approaches to life. Everyone develops a characteristic "explanatory style," according to Seligman.

When something bad happens to a person with a pessimistic explanatory style, that person often accepts total blame and sees the event as part of a long-term pattern of failure. An optimistic person will shrug off the event as temporary and perhaps due to extenuating circumstances. If you lost your house keys on the way home from work, for example, you might explain it by saying, "I'm always losing everything because I am careless, and I will always lose things in this way." Or you might say, "I lost my house keys because I was preoccupied with that big deal at work." One explanation is characteristic of the pessimist, the other of the optimist. An optimist also is more likely to assume that anything good that happens is due to his or her character rather than to a one-time lightning bolt of luck. This is not to say that the optimist never assumes blame for anything or is never sad or depressed. Everybody makes mistakes and experiences sadness, guilt, and worry. But, overall, the person who views life optimistically is more likely to expect success and to see failure as a temporary setback.

Can such differences in outlook really affect our health and the likelihood of getting a disease? Between 1939 and 1944, two hundred Harvard College freshmen were selected for a lifelong study of health and success. For the last half century these men—some of them now prominent figures—have cheerfully submitted to physical exams, interviews, and questionnaires. In the 1980s, Seligman used this group to study the relationship between optimism and long-term health.

Seligman and his fellow researchers analyzed ninety-nine randomly selected essays written by the Harvard men in 1945–46 after they had served in the military during World War II. The researchers had no idea who these men were and knew nothing of their health histories, their financial success, who had lived and who had died. All their knowledge was gathered from the essays. Two men said, for example, that they had been unhappy with their military work and

responsibilities, but for very different reasons. The more optimistic man had been discouraged because "many things were left undone in the press of circumstances." The more pessimistic man cited "an intrinsic dislike for the military." From many hundreds of such statements, the researchers assembled a picture of their ninety-nine subjects as they were as young men returning from war. Only then did they review the health file of each man, looking for correlations between optimism and health. "What we saw was that health at age sixty was strongly related to optimism at age twenty-five," Seligman wrote. The researchers found no correlation between health and optimism until the Harvard men reached about age forty-five. From that point on, the more pessimistic men got sick sooner, and more severely, with the characteristic diseases of middle age.

Another study sent Seligman's researchers to the newspaper sports pages, where they reviewed fifty years of quotations from famous baseball players who eventually made it into the Baseball Hall of Fame. Correlating the quotes with health and mortality data from public record, the researchers found that ballplayers who pessimistically blamed themselves in defeat were younger when they died and were more likely to have been sick than those who did not blame themselves for losses.

The Tie That Binds for Health

If there were a single prescription a doctor could write for a young man or woman to encourage a lifetime of good health, it might be this: "Keep other people close to you. Seek their support, and support them in return." Four out of the top five items on the Holmes-Rahe scale of stressful life events involve the loss of close relationships and social support. Among the pioneer studies of mind-body health were those that noted premature deaths among those who had recently lost a spouse through death. More recently, researchers have discovered that the hopelessness and depression that accompany such losses can precipitate measurable decreases in immune function. Based on such observations, researchers have long suspected that close, supporting relationships encourage health—that to the "three Cs" of hardiness should be added a fourth: connectedness.

But how do you measure the importance of connectedness in a large group of people? In the mid-1970s, psychologist Lisa Berkman reviewed a set of ten-year-old questionnaires on the lifestyles and social relationships of nearly seven thousand Californians. Berkman divided her subjects into two groups—an isolated group, in which people had reported having few social and community ties, and a supported group, of people who reported such connections. On the basis of death certificates filed with the California health department, Berkman concluded that the isolated, lonely people were dying at more than twice the rate of their more socially connected peers.

Other research has examined the effects on health when traditionally cohesive groups are disrupted. The Japanese, for example, have traditionally enjoyed some of the best health in the world, including a rate of heart disease one-fifth that of Americans. After immigrating to America, some Japanese families move toward a more typically American pattern of heart disease, as succeeding generations adopt a new way of life. Other Japanese-Americans maintain the superior health of those in their homeland—despite a diet rich in fats; crowded, polluted cities; and a rapid pace of life. Studies by Dr. Leonard Syme, an epidemiologist at the University of California, Berkeley, and his associates suggest that one critical difference between these two groups may be their social cohesion and support.

In traditional Japanese culture, the individual is entangled in an interwoven fabric of commitment, responsibility, and support and can spend a lifetime interacting with the same people at home, school, and work. The Japanese concept of *amae* expresses a belief that the well-being of the individual depends on the cooperation of others and the goodwill of the group. Dr. Syme and the other researchers found that members of Japanese families who retained this spirit of group interconnectedness after immigrating to the United States also retained the superior pattern of health. No other variable explained the differing levels of heart disease between the two groups—not genetics, sex, social class, age, cholesterol level,

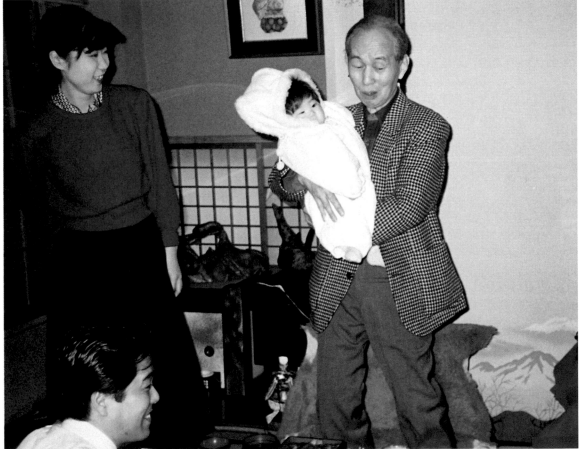

The Japanese concept of *amae* expresses the interconnectedness of the individual with family members and society. Some researchers believe that these close relationships may account, in part, for the high standard of Japanese health.

cigarette smoking, or blood pressure. The key to the health of these people was the support of their families and friends.

What kind of social support is important? The support of bosses and co-workers has been linked to increased resistance to a number of diseases, including rashes, ulcers, heart disease, and chronic lung conditions. Long-term, committed partnerships, such as marriage, seem particularly crucial—especially for men. In Berkman's study of nearly seven thousand Californians, unmarried men between the ages of thirty and sixty years were two to three times as likely to die as their married peers. A study by researchers at Duke University, published in the *Journal of the American Medical Association*, found that heart disease patients were three times as likely to die within five years of diagnosis if they had no spouse or good friend in whom to confide.

Cancer, heart disease, arthritis, depression, tuberculosis, and problems of pregnancy all occur more frequently in people with weakened social support. One reason may be that people undoubtedly have better health habits when others value and depend on them for support. Close friends and relatives may also provide help in the form of money or physical assistance in times of crisis, which may provide a greater feeling of control over stressful circumstances.

Studies have found that loneliness also can work directly on the immune system. A study of medical students at Ohio State University found that the number of natural killer cells decreased in most students faced with the stress of exams but that the loneliest students experienced the largest decreases. Another study found that healthy elderly people with close relationships have better immune function and lower levels of cholesterol than healthy elderly people without such relationships. In some way, our bodies seem to need the solace and support of human communication and companionship.

Personality, Meaning, and Health
In recent years Americans have been besieged with information on what their bodies need for health. It seems as though every issue of the morning newspaper carries a new warning or exhortation: Avoid saturated fats, don't smoke cigarettes, eat your broccoli, get the right amount of the right kind of exercise and sleep. Sometimes these rapidly accumulating rules seem like a recipe for health to which the doctors are continually adding new ingredients. By following these rules, we hope to earn seven or eight decades of relative health in which to raise a family, pursue a career, acquire friends and lovers, learn what we wish to learn, and go where we wish to go. In this traditional view, good health is a goal that when achieved makes it possible for us to enjoy the important parts of our lives.

One of the important messages of the new mind-body research is that good health is more than following rules—it does not simply *make possible* the living of our lives but emerges *from* the living of our lives. Health emerges from hope, optimism, laughter, connectedness, support, commitment, self-worth, a sense of control, and perhaps something more: the perception that life has meaning and that each of us has some unique role that cannot be played by anyone else. At the same time, these forces for health should not be thought of as emotional and interpersonal inoculations against disease. We all know of people who became sick and died young even though their lives overflowed with love, commitment, humor, and self-worth. No one experiences such emotions, however, without being in some way healthier in the word's root sense of "whole," "wholesome," and "holy."

This larger notion of health includes but is not limited to physical health or mental health, for even together the two concepts do not necessarily incorporate the importance of meaning, purpose, and wholesome balance. According to the larger definition, no one who perceives life as meaningless is truly healthy, no matter how lengthy and disease-free the person's life may be, and anyone who finds meaning and purpose in life will remain in some sense healthy through physical decline and death. The emerging mind-body science seems to carry both a hopeful message and a warning. The message: What most enriches our lives is also good for our health. The warning: No society can grow healthy individuals if it does not foster personal hope, optimism, commitment, and self-worth.

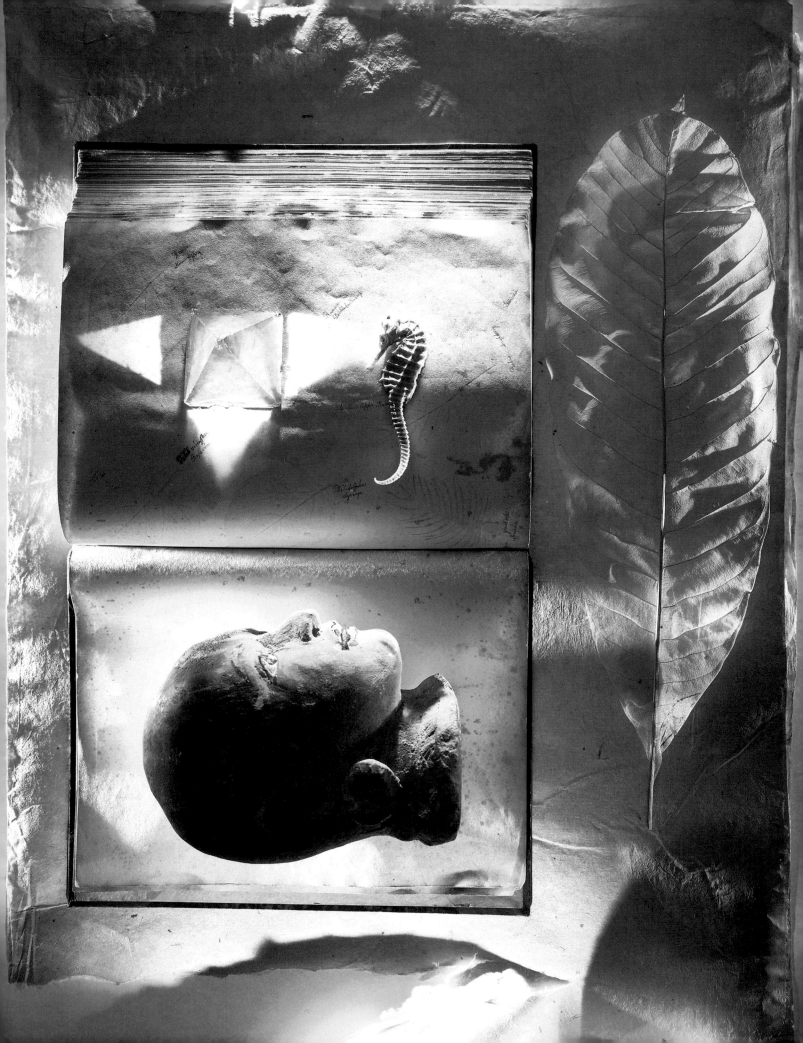

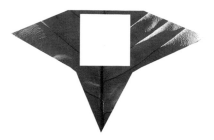

CHAPTER FIVE

GETTING WELL

A CASEBOOK OF HEALING TECHNIQUES

A NEW INTEREST IN THERAPIES

IN 1992, THE NATIONAL INSTITUTES of Health established a special office to support research into "alternative" medical treatments. It was a big step, for federal funding had rarely been used to support research outside the medical mainstream. Treatments targeted for possible study included those based on psychological interventions and specific mind-body control techniques.

What is driving the government's new interest in mind-body therapies? Much of the pressure comes from a public growing increasingly disenchanted with the cost, complexity, and impersonality of mainstream medicine. As scientists unravel the basic connections between mind and body, both the public and its legislators are eager to explore the field's practical implications. Can people really change personality traits that might make them ill? Can people "think themselves well" through meditation or by picturing themselves as healthy? Can relatively simple mind-body therapies gradually reduce the need for expensive technological medicine?

These are not easy questions, and the new federally sponsored research may help find more answers.

> *"Natural forces within us are the true healers of disease."*
>
> —HIPPOCRATES

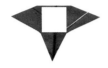

But evidence has long been accumulating that such specific mind-body tools as meditation, visualization, and biofeedback can reduce stress, produce health-promoting relaxation, and alter specific bodily processes. Other therapies have been shown to help people cope with stress, promote personal control, and increase optimism, thus preserving and restoring health and balance. Some of these techniques and therapies are extensions of ancient healing or religious practices, while others are based on the very latest microprocessor wizardry. All assume the mind has a degree of influence on bodily processes that scientists would have thought impossible only a few decades ago.

Learning to Relax

The Dorchester section of Boston is a poor, inner-city neighborhood with the attendant ills. There are guns and violence and gangs. At Dorchester High School, students may arrive at their classrooms bearing books, homework, and more than a little stress. Like all teenagers, they face family conflicts, peer-group tensions, and questions about the future. But the teachers at Dorchester High like to think they've created a refuge for their students, and work hard to supply them with tools for life. One day recently, a circle of Dorchester High faculty sat in the school library, eyes closed in deep relaxation.

"Either close or lower your eyes," suggests Dr. Olivia Hoblitzelle, an instructor from the Mind/Body Medical Institute at New England Deaconess Hospital. "You're turning your attention deep inside. Take several slow, long, deep breaths. As you breathe in, begin to calm your body and your mind. As you breathe out, very consciously begin to let go of any physical tensions, any worries, any preoccupations, so you're being very present with your breath."

Hoblitzelle asks members of the group if they have noticed any changes.

"My arms are heavy," responds one teacher.

"I feel totally calm and focused on the moment."

"I forgot that I was in the room."

The technique helps people relax and manage stress, Hoblitzelle tells the teachers. It will help their students learn to concentrate, a skill essential for study and life. It will also help them create an inner calm. By learning to stay the rush of outer anxieties, they will gain awareness and control regardless of the exact circumstances of their lives. "Only with awareness," she says, "do you have choice."

The Dorchester High program is a reminder of how far we have come since researchers and therapists first became interested in deep physiological relaxation in the early decades of this century. Even as scientists were outlining the body's fight-or-flight response to stress, other researchers were wondering how the response might be switched off—reducing blood pressure, heart rate, breathing rate, and muscular tension, and so restoring relaxation and calm.

Earlier in this century, several doctors proposed relaxation techniques based on the mental control of muscular tension and bodily processes. Typically, subjects were instructed to lie or sit quietly and to progressively relax their muscles, slow their breathing and heart rate, and imagine calming sensations. Then, in 1975, a Harvard cardiologist named Herbert Benson announced that he had measured profound relaxation in subjects during transcendental meditation, or TM, a form of Eastern meditation that was gaining prominence in the West. Like many "discoveries" of mind-body medicine, this was, in fact, a rediscovery of ancient and widely held beliefs about healing. Meditational exercises are part of many religious traditions and help produce the rewarding serenity some people gain from spiritual observance. The association of meditation and health is also a deep one. The word *meditation* comes from the Latin *meditari*, meaning "to think about, to consider," and is related to the Latin root for medicine, *mederi*, which means "to heal or look after." In turn, both words are thought to spring from the ancient Indo-European root *med*, meaning "to take appropriate measures."

Dr. Joan Borysenko, a former director of the Mind/Body Clinic at New England Deaconess Hospital, defines meditation as "the capacity to absorb ourselves in the present moment," what is sometimes called "mindfulness." She believes the process heals not only physically but emotionally and spiritually. The physical benefits come from the relaxation response, the tuning down of the body's stress. Emotionally, meditation decreases anxiety and calms the mind. Spiritual benefits descend from what Borysenko calls "a sense of edgelessness. . . . We lose our boundaries and feel at one with something larger than ourselves."

Whether pursued simply for relaxation, or for spiritual enlightenment or healing, meditation requires a quiet, comfortable setting; a conscious effort to relax the muscles, regulate the breathing, and calm the mind; and a device to facilitate mental focusing. A special word, called a mantra, or a meaningful religious phrase may be used to focus attention, or the mind may be directed toward mental images of calming scenes or to the simple rhythm of breathing. TM is similar to many meditative practices

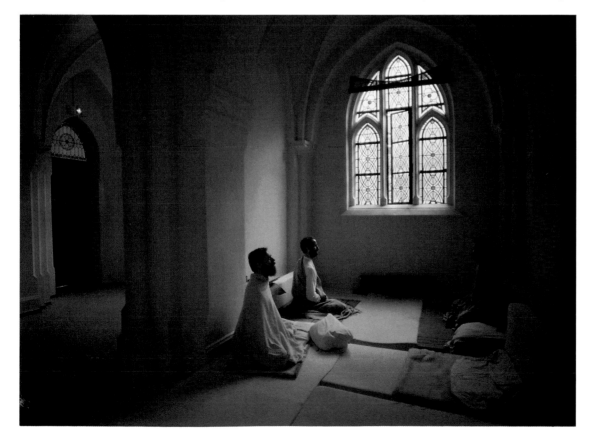

Meditation has been practiced for thousands of years, by people in search of spritual enlightenment and deep physical and mental calm.

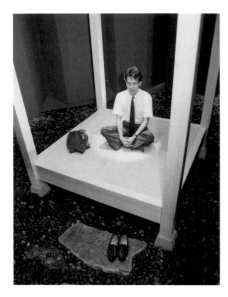

Meditation has been found to produce a physiological state different from both simple rest and sleep. This meditation room, in a Tokyo office building, offers workers a break from daily stress.

of the Hindu, Buddhist, and Taoist traditions. New students of TM are told to sit in a comfortable position in a quiet place and to concentrate for about twenty minutes on their mantra, so that extraneous thoughts and worries can pass through the mind unattended.

The TM movement was part of an interest in Eastern religious practices that swept sections of the country in the 1960s and 1970s and still continues today. Prominent TM students of the 1970s included actress Mia Farrow and members of the Beatles. Practiced properly and regularly, TM was said to lead to an expanding sense of consciousness and a perception of oneness with creation. With the mind stilled, the body could achieve deep relaxation and a transforming calm.

Hoping to obtain a scientific measure of the effects of TM on the body, in the early 1970s the movement's proponents asked Dr. Benson and another researcher, R. Keith Wallace, to monitor meditators for physiological change. The scientists wired their subjects with electrodes and drew blood samples before and after meditation. What they discovered confirmed that the calm felt by TM practitioners was definitely not "all in their minds" but a unique physiological state distinct from either simple rest or sleep. It was as if the fight-or-flight response were shifted into reverse. Heart and breathing rates and blood pressure went down, as did the rate at which meditators consumed oxygen. Moreover, this physiological calm occurred whithin minutes. TM seemed like an ever-ready antidote to the health-eroding stress of modern life.

From here, Dr. Benson and fellow researcher Wallace parted company. Wallace was a TM practitioner himself and was convinced that some transcendental process unique to TM produced the deep, physiological calm. Benson, by contrast, sought to strip meditation of its religious trappings. What was important, he suggested, was the act of quiet concentration. Benson termed the resulting physiological reaction "the relaxation response." This was also the title of his 1976 book, which became a bestseller and a major influence on a generation of health practitioners.

In the years since Benson's and Wallace's pioneering work, meditation and "relaxation exercises" have become the most common techniques for helping the mind combat stress and promote concentration. Critical to the process is the ability to focus the mind, to exclude the barrage of thoughts, worries, and preoccupations that bombard our consciousness from within and without. Such mental exercises are a variety of self-hypnosis, a courting of the altered state of consciousness long associated with healing.

In health-care settings, relaxation and meditation exercises often are employed for the relief of stress and anxiety and for the management of chronic pain, all of which are bound together in an inextricable knot. Some clinical psychologists use meditation to help clients cleanse their minds of tensions and everyday worries before individual or group psychotherapy sessions. Relaxation has also been shown to improve immune function, probably because it prevents the release of immune-reducing fight-or-flight stress chemicals. For this reason, the technique has been used to treat everything from colds to AIDS. Some people who have achieved spontaneous remissions of cancer claim to have done so in part through intensive meditation. Just as important, the ability to achieve a relaxed mental state is a skill for life, as Hoblitzelle tells the teachers at Dorchester High. Who would not welcome a sense of calm, focus, self-mastery, and inner control? "That is an important gift to give any youngster," she says, "to say nothing of ourselves."

Visualizing a Cure

In 1982, when Doris Phillips was fifty-six, her physician, James Suen of the University of Arkansas Medical Center, suggested chemotherapy for her throat cancer, which had recently spread to Phillips's lungs. Dr. Suen, a prominent throat specialist, who has also treated President Bill Clinton's recurring laryngitis, had little hope for Phillips. Over the previous twenty years, she had endured two major surgeries and thirty radiation treatments for adenocystic carcinoma, a slow-growing but inexorably recurring form of cancer. The chemotherapy might temporarily shrink the suffocating tumors in Phillips's lungs, he told her, but it would not cure her. She decided not to undergo the chemotherapy, to set her affairs in order, and to prepare to die.

In the meantime, overwhelming depression led Phillips to a counselor, who presented her with a book about cancer recovery, *Getting Well Again*, by Carl and Stephanie Simonton. The Simontons recommended, as an adjunct to standard cancer therapies, a program of relaxation, attitude change, and mental imaging. In particular, they suggested that patients form a mental picture of their cancer and of the immune system's victory over the disease.

Such techniques are based on the ancient notion that a picture or image held in the mind can effect bodily change. Our minds are inexhaustible storehouses of images, and accumulating evidence suggests that, under the right conditions, these images may work their way into the nervous system, into the immune system, into our organs, muscles, sinews, and

bones. Psychologists have long recognized that images are preverbal, deeply linked to our emotions and unconscious mind, and therefore able to reflect feelings and internal states that we are unable to put into words or thoughts. The interpretation of dreams is based on this psychological truth. Artists also have recognized that images can communicate feelings in ways our thinking minds cannot understand. Whenever we say that a painting, a photograph, a piece of music, or the smell of a flower moves us in a way we cannot express, we are acknowledging the power of images.

The parts of our brain that create and respond to images may be the same parts that enable healing to take place and our bodies to maintain health. The placebo effect partly results from a patient's positive mental images concerning treatment and cure, and much of the extraordinary healing discussed in this book may depend on mental images. Remember the story about the woman in the hypnotic trance who broke out into a sunburn after being told to picture herself on the beach? Such bodily changes under hypnosis are mental images made flesh.

Images are also central to shamanistic healing. A shaman often diagnoses disease by interpreting images from dreams or visions. In telling stories about the origin and cure of a patient's disease, the shaman creates a vivid picture for the patient of illness and cure within a spiritual and cultural context. In the Western tradition, for centuries after the rise of Greek medicine, diagnosis was based on the interpretation of dream images. Contemporary uses of imagery build upon these older traditions. In therapeutic imagery—sometimes called visualization, although it is not always a visual image that is created—a person might construct an image that relates directly to the physiology of the disease. To heal a skin disease, for example, the person might hold an image of cleansing in the mind. To help knit a broken bone, a person might concentrate on an image of the bone marrow flowing from one side of the break to the other. Although some therapists report success with such treatments, especially on highly hypnotizable people, organized studies have yet to be done.

By far the most high-profile and controversial use of imagery has been in the treatment of cancer. The

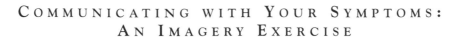

The next time you are sick, you might want to try the following imagery exercise to promote healing. The exercise comes from Dr. Marty Rossman, co-director of the Academy for Guided Imagery in Mill Valley, California. The purpose of the exercise is to create a helpful, healing relationship with the symptoms of your illness. Most of us, whether we realize it or not, automatically think of a symptom as an adversary and a nuisance, but much can be learned from taking a new look at a symptom by calling up its image. Remember, images are not only visual. Try to find out also how the symptom sounds, smells, tastes, and feels. Entering into a "dialogue" with a symptom may reveal something of its meaning to you and help you uncover previously unconscious feelings. The goal is not necessarily to "cure," but to encourage peace of mind and healing.

- 1. Begin by relaxing, and then focus directly on the symptom. Allow yourself to accept whatever image comes, whether it seems right or not, whether it is expected or not, whether you like it or not. (The image might make sense to you—for example, a knife might appear as an image for pain—but the image might not make sense. Remember, the image does not come from your "thinking self" but from your unconscious.)

- 2. Explore the image for a while. Observe it in as much detail as possible. Move around it. Get inside it. What features draw your attention? How far away or how close is it? How big is it? How big is it in relation to you? (By answering these questions, you may begin to reframe your relationship to that image.)

- 3. What qualities does this image convey to you? (Every image is alive and can communicate with you. Imagine that you can communicate back.)

- 4. What feelings do you have as you observe the image? (This question may be repeated several times, since the feelings one has about illness may be complex. Examining these feelings may enable deeper feelings to emerge—for example, pity toward the image, rather than anger at its existence. Let yourself be honest about your feelings and how they come up.)

- 5. Now express those feelings—all of them—directly toward the image.

- 6. Imagine the image can answer back—give voice to the image, and let it answer you. Listen and observe carefully. Let the image respond. (The image tends to come to life at this point.) After a while, you can begin to ask the image these and other questions: "Why are you here?" (Let it answer.) What do you want from me? How do you function in me? What do you need from me? What are you trying to do for me?

- 7. Explore what it's like to be the image—to be that part of yourself. What does the world look like as you look out through the image's eyes? What does it feel like to be that image? (At this point, you will probably begin to develop some empathy for that part of yourself.)

- 8. Now look at the image again from your own perspective. Does it look the same or different? Have you learned anything about it that you didn't know before?

- 9. Continue communicating with the image. Do you feel willing to give it what it wants or needs? (What we're trying to do is open up the lines of communication and learn how to live in greater harmony with each element of ourselves.)

- 10. When you feel the process is complete, gradually bring yourself back to the everyday world and review what you have learned.

Simontons and others suggest that the use of the right kind of imagery can directly stimulate the immune system, strengthening the body against the effects of growth or the recurrence of a tumor. Though highly controversial, this argument is supported by experiments in which some subjects were able to increase various immune measures through visualization exercises.

For her part, Doris Phillips decided she had little to lose in following the advice in the Simontons' book. Several times each day she would retreat to the quiet of her bedroom, relax, and start talking to her body. Phillips's daughter Aven, a nurse, provided her mother with a normal chest x-ray and pictures of immune cells devouring cancer cells. Phillips also studied her own chest x-ray, to fix in her mind the locations of her tumors. Phillips pictured the war going on in her body as a Pac-Man video game in which her immune cells were gobbling her cancer cells. "I would call on all my good cells to come and eat the cancer cells away," she would later write. "I explained to my good cells that the cancer cells were parasites trying to rob us of our bodily home." At the same time, Phillips assumed a new attitude toward her disease. She called her children to announce she had decided not to die. "I quit being happy with my illness," Phillips remembered. "I quit calling it 'my cancer.' Of course it was hard in the beginning. I missed seeing the sad looks on people's faces when I told them I had cancer. If the subject did come up I would say, 'Back when I had cancer.' "

When Phillips went for her regular checkup a few months later, she was sure she was getting better and was at first discouraged when Dr. Suen announced that she was simply no worse. "I'll just have to work harder," Phillips decided. Doubling her imaging efforts, she would disappear into her bedroom four or five times each day. At no time over those months did she mention to Dr. Suen what she was doing. By the time of the next checkup, Phillips was convinced that she was well and eagerly awaited Dr. Suen's verification. When the doctor entered the room, Phillips knew he had seen her x-rays. "He came in with a strange look on his face," she recalled. "He asked me what I had been doing and showed me that the tumors were all gone. He asked a million questions." A decade later, Phillips is still well.

"Flabbergasted" is the word Dr. Suen used to describe his reactions to Phillips's x-rays—he had never heard of a complete remission from Phillips's type of cancer. "For a long time I never brought up this case to other people," Suen said. "I thought maybe it was a fluke." Then, by coincidence, Suen encountered psychologist Stephanie Simonton, whose book had begun Phillips's journey of self-healing and who had recently moved her practice to Arkansas. Simonton told Suen that although Phillips might be an unusual self-healer, her case was probably not a fluke. Simonton wanted to do controlled research on the effect of imagery in cancer patients, and, in light of Doris Phillips's case, Dr. Suen decided it would be a good idea.

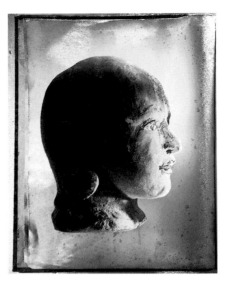

"The power of people doing things for themselves is very strong medicine."

—KATE LORIG, NURSE

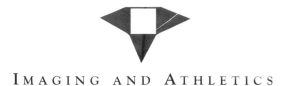

Two months before the 1984 Summer Olympic Games in Los Angeles, a Romanian weight lifter named Dragomir Cioroslan fell backward during a lift and dropped a six-hundred-pound barbell across his neck. For ten days he could not stand, and it would be weeks before he'd return to the gym.

The accident could have been the end of Cioroslan's dramatic and unlikely athletic career. As a child, he had suffered from rheumatic heart disease, rheumatoid arthritis, and chronic bronchitis. When he began weight lifting, at fifteen, he weighed only seventy pounds and couldn't even lift the twenty-five-pound bar to which weights are fastened. At the time of his accident, Cioroslan was already a world champion weight lifter, but his greatest dream was to win an Olympic medal. After his accident, that dream seemed to be over. "I couldn't move, couldn't train, and almost saw my dream falling apart," Cioroslan remembers. "I was devastated. I didn't know what to do. I

asked for any advice I could have." That advice came to him from his sports psychologist. "Visualize," he was told, "continue your training in your mind."

So, while his fellow hospital patients dozed or paged through magazines, Cioroslan closed his eyes and worked, eight hours a day, every day. "I started to imagine, to recreate in my mind every movement I did in the gym, from strapping my belt around my lower back to the heaviest lift over my head. For every detail of my movements—with light weights, intermediates, heavy weights—I went through the same feelings, through the same movements, trying to visualize and recreate those images again and again."

When he finally got back to the weight room, Cioroslan discovered that every minute of his unconventional training had been worthwhile. Not only had he improved his powers of concentration and visualization, but he had burned into his mind the image of a winning

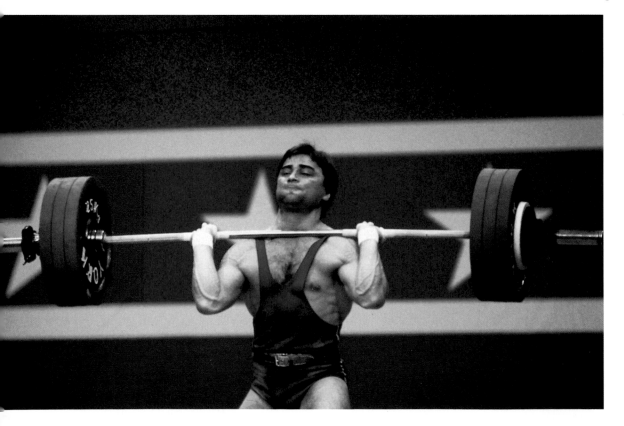

Using concentration and visualization techniques, Romanian weight lifter Cioroslan Dragomir recovered rapidly from an injury, competed in the 1984 Olympic Summer Games in Los Angeles, and won a bronze medal.

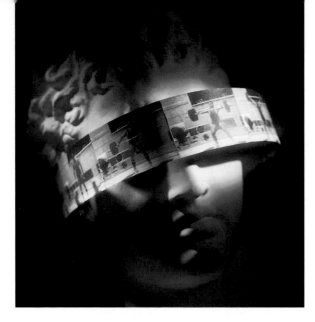

form. He came back from his injury more quickly than he had ever anticipated. After only two weeks of training, he competed in the Olympics in Los Angeles, where he stood on the winners' podium, a bronze medal around his neck.

Cioroslan's story confirms what every skilled athlete understands: no sports accomplishment is purely physical. Athletic excellence demands mental toughness, single-minded dedication, immense concentration, an appropriate degree of relaxation and self-confidence, and an ability to imagine success and to picture the steps of a perfect dive or high jump or home run. Because relaxation is crucial, many athletes rely on meditation and other relaxation techniques to loosen up before an event. Biofeedback training offers one way to measure relaxation and to learn to control tension-producing bodily processes. One frequently used portable device measures skin perspiration, an indication of stress. The goal for an athlete may not be total relaxation, but to learn — and to be able to duplicate — exactly the amount of internal stress needed to perform at peak capacity.

The most important mind-body tool for any athlete may be imagery and visualization. Former Olympic pentathlete Marilyn King, who coaches people on the use of imagery in sports and other activities, says athletes rely on mental images "to envision both a goal and the steps to achieving it." King herself suffered an injury before the 1980 Olympic trials and spent four bedridden months watching films of the world's best pentathletes and imagining her own body performing at that level.

During competition, athletes use imagery to focus inward, to center their attention and eliminate outside distractions. They make "mental movies" of successfully completing a task, whether it be fielding a grounder, throwing a pass, or shooting a basket. As athletes improve, they assemble an internal library of images associated with peak performance. Duplicating that performance often depends as much on reproducing those images — rerunning those mental movies — as it does on the athlete's physical strength and conditioning. The athlete relies on three kinds of mental imagery, King says: visual, kinetic (the feeling of the body in motion), and auditory — usually in combination. "For example, as you are standing on the long-jump runway at the beginning of the event, you *see* yourself accelerating, you feel the wind resistance, and you hear your footsteps as you accelerate."

Also important is the athlete's internal image that the ultimate goals can be accomplished. King points out that before 1954 it was widely believed that a human was physically incapable of running a mile in less than four minutes. That year, British runner Roger Bannister proved the skeptics wrong, showing long-distance runners worldwide that the feat could be accomplished. Within twelve months, fifty-two other athletes had run miles in less than four minutes, overcoming what had been a *psychological* rather than a *physiological* barrier.

The principles of imaging clearly have applications outside sports, King maintains. "For me the value in coaching doesn't lie in creating a stable of seven-foot, six-inch-high jumpers, but in showing athletes that the first step toward stunning achievement is believing that you can do it. Most people need to understand that once you dare to imagine something, you begin to be flooded with ideas of how to realize that image."

Suen brought Simonton and Phillips together, and on May 23, 1984, the doctor, the psychologist, and the woman who believed she'd healed herself of cancer presented her case to a group of extremely attentive local cancer doctors. That meeting, and others that followed, ultimately led to a new program of psychological research and support at the Arkansas Cancer Research Center, and Stephanie Simonton has begun a National Cancer Institute–supported study of the effect of imaging on adenocystic carcinoma. The inexplicable and well-documented cure of Doris Phillips helped convince the NCI that such a study might be worth conducting.

Biofeedback: Technology for the Mind's Eye

At Jackson Memorial Medical Center in Miami, a twelve-year-old boy with a mop of blond hair and a big smile shuffles into the hospital's Biofeedback and Electrical Stimulation Laboratory. Chris Kelly was never expected to be able to walk at all—even with the aid of the walker he is using today. Deprived of oxygen at birth, the cells in Chris's brain that controlled these actions died. The boy spent much of his early life in a wheelchair. Now, thanks to Dr. Bernard Brucker and a laboratory full of electronic gear, Chris may soon be walking with a cane, leaving both walker and wheelchair behind.

Brucker, the laboratory's director, is not a physical therapist: He does not help patients restore function and build muscles through exercise. He is a psychologist and biofeedback therapist who uses technology to help people glimpse the action of their own brains—and retrain those brains to accomplish bodily tasks. Brucker fastens electrodes to Chris's ankles and lower legs and attaches these to a computer and video screen. The computer measures the electrical impulse transmitted to the muscles from Chris's brain, and the biofeedback apparatus enables Chris to see these impulses as colored lines on the video screen. By mentally increasing one impulse at a time—by adjusting the movement of the lines on the screen—he is learning to manipulate his ankle in a walking movement. To Chris, it's a little like playing a video game, but for higher stakes. "Bring that blue line up a little bit more," Brucker encourages the boy. "Good, good. Now keep that yellow line down."

For a long time, Western medicine has assumed that what Chris Kelly is attempting is impossible. Brain and spinal cord injuries have been thought to be permanent, for the simple reason that damaged nerves do not regenerate. Physicians have assumed that specific bodily motions are irrevocably assigned to specific nerve cells and that when these nerves die so does the ability to move. Brucker and other scientists are demonstrating that our bodies and brains are more flexible than this. (Researchers frequently use the word *plastic* to refer to this flexibility, meaning, roughly, "capable of change.")

According to Brucker, any brain or spinal cord cells that remain, regardless of their original function, can often be retrained to carry the impulses needed to take a step, for example, or to lift a coffee cup. Since 1981, the biofeedback laboratory at Jackson Memorial has treated more than two thousand people suffering from paralysis or other motion disabilities. In 90 percent, functioning has improved, and more than a dozen totally incapacitated patients have been able to restore most of their mobility.

How do people make such remarkable improvements? What goes on in Chris Kelly's mind as he retrains his nerves to assume new roles? Is it like learning to ride a bicycle or drive a car? The brain learns which signal, out of hundreds of signals, will increase or decrease the lines on the screen and make a foot inch forward. Somehow the boy "thinks" the physical impulse that makes the movement happen.

While Brucker is breaking new ground in using biofeedback to rehabilitate victims of crippling brain and spinal cord injuries, biofeedback techniques have been used for nearly fifty years—for as long as the technology has been available. Early mind-body researchers understood that it is easier for the mind to regulate and control bodily processes if changes are easily and instantly observed. It is much easier to learn relaxation techniques, for example, if the physiological signs of relaxation—such as decreasing heart rate, blood pressure, and sweating—are "fed back" to the subject in the form of lines on a screen or a tone in a headset. Under these conditions, one can learn to relax in the same way one learns to drive a car or shoot a basketball: through trial and error.

Biofeedback developed from animal experiments in

the 1940s and 1950s, in which rats learned to alter their heart rate and blood pressure to get food. By the 1960s, humans were being wired to electronic gear to help them control bodily and mental processes. Much attention was focused on so-called alpha training, which enables some people to regulate the patterns of their brain waves to produce relaxation or other states of consciousness. Biofeedback thus became associated in the public mind with the consciousness-expanding movement of the 1970s, and some people continue to think of it as a kind of counterculture fad. In the last decade, however, biofeedback has quietly blossomed into one of our most powerful mind-body treatments, and more than a hundred biofeedback devices are now in use. Most commonly, they measure blood pressure, heart rate, muscle tension, or the temperature and chemistry of the skin.

The renaissance of biofeedback in the last decade has depended on achievements in two key areas. First, neuroscientists have increased our knowledge of the way the brain controls the body. Second, advances in computers and miniaturization have made possible faster and more sophisticated monitoring of bodily functions. As we gain knowledge in both these areas, biofeedback promises to become one of the primary tools for helping the mind manage health. Alone or in combination with relaxation therapy, biofeedback training has been used to treat migraine

Spurred by recent advances in neuroscience and technology, biofeedback techniques allow people to visualize internal processes so they can be controlled through trial-and-error learning. Finger temperature and the degree of sweating provide measurements of bodily relaxation.

Other techniques allow the study of the various frequencies of brain waves associated with thought, relaxation, and creativity. By recording and later reviewing brain-wave activity, a person can work to create a calm or creative mind-body state.

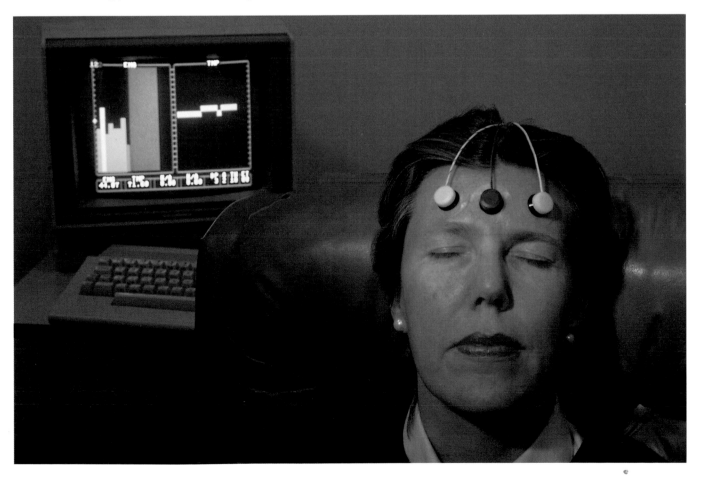

Opposite page: NASA scientists have been using biofeedback to help astronauts control the motion sickness associated with weightlessness. Sensors built into a special space suit measure heart rate, respiratory rate, and movement of the head, while a wristwatch-like display reads out the data. By being aware of these bodily processes, an astronaut can use mental techniques to control them. Shown is Mae Jemison, the United States's first black woman astronaut, who wore the biofeedback device in space.

headaches, high blood pressure, low blood pressure, and diabetes and to restore bladder control to patients suffering from urinary incontinence. Biofeedback is the only treatment for a rare condition called Raynaud's disease, in which there is insufficient circulation of blood to the hands and feet, leading to ulcers or serious infection.

The National Aeronautics and Space Administration (NASA) is even testing biofeedback in space. Astronauts are frequently plagued with "space adaptation syndrome," a form of motion sickness that results from weightlessness. In the absence of gravity, the inner ear has difficulty controlling the sense of balance, producing nausea. Some astronauts vomit for the first several days in space, while others seek relief with medication that may make them sleepy and disoriented. In response, NASA has launched a test program to see if astronauts can learn to control space sickness through biofeedback training. On the ground, the effects of weightlessness are simulated in a rotating chair and in an experimental jet aircraft the astronauts have affectionately nicknamed "the vomit comet." This modified KC-135, which flies straight up, straight down, and in looping parabolas, can produce weightlessness for as long as twenty seconds.

While they're in the KC-135, the astronauts wear a biofeedback body suit. A ring worn on a finger measures each astronaut's skin temperature and the amount of blood flowing to the hands. Other electrodes, in the sleeve of the suit, measure heart rate, respiratory rate, and the movement of the head. A display similar to a wristwatch provides a constant readout of these physiological responses, while a data recorder on the belt of the suit records the responses for future study. Biofeedback training teaches astronauts how they react to the stress of weightlessness, as well as mental techniques for controlling space sickness. Early tests in space suggest that the technique may one day work as well for some astronauts as drugs do, without the disorienting side effects.

Another promising area in biofeedback research is brain-wave training, a descendant of the alpha training of the 1960s. In measuring the electrical activity of the brain, scientists have associated different mental states with brain waves of different lengths: alpha waves, which predominate during relaxation; beta waves, which seem associated with thinking; and theta waves, which seem present during daydreaming, imagery, and creative visualization. During brain-wave training, a subject monitors his or her own brain-wave changes through a graphic representation on a monitor or a tone in a headset. Subjects working toward a more creative, imaginative state might strive to increase the number of theta waves, while those learning to relax might use the proportion of alpha waves as a guide to their progress.

In 1989, psychologist Eugene Peniston created a stir in the professional biofeedback community by announcing that alpha-theta brain-wave training seemed remarkably effective in treating chronic alcoholics. Through brain-wave training, Peniston reasoned, alcoholics could

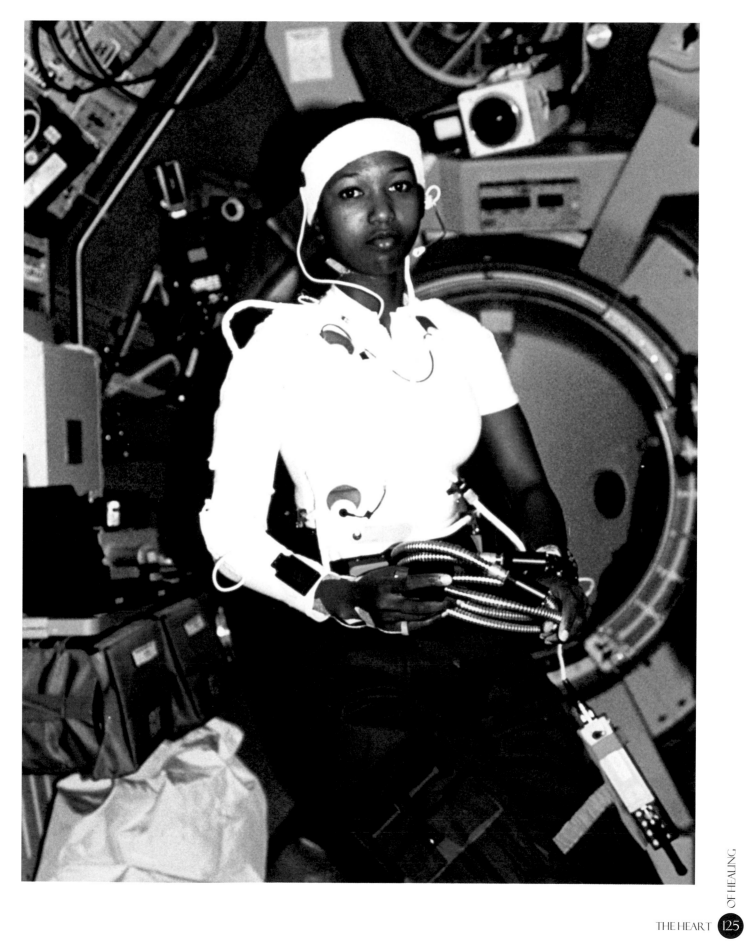

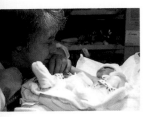

In the neonatal intensive care unit at Stanford Children's Hospital in California, a nurse approaches an isolette—a covered, plastic crib—containing a sleeping baby. The nurse has not come to give the premature infant medicine, or to adjust its intravenous fluids or breathing tube, or to check the bank of monitors that measures everything from the baby's heart rate to the oxygen concentration in its blood. She has come instead to apply a treatment as old has healing itself, a modern version of the ancient "laying on of hands."

Her face grows calm as she inserts her hands through two portholes in the walls of the isolette. Cupping one hand above the baby's head, she slowly sweeps the other hand down the baby's body, above the surface of the blanket. The nurses at Stanford have found that premature babies receiving such "therapeutic touch" treatments seem calmer afterward and oxygenate their bodies better. These nurses are not alone in their assessment. Since the treatment was pioneered by Dolores Krieger, a nurse, in the mid-1970s, therapeutic touch has developed a growing following among the nation's nurses. Today, an estimated twenty thousand to thirty thousand nurses incorporate therapeutic touch into their routine care of children and adults.

Like some other treatments that are labeled "alternative," therapeutic touch is based on assumptions foreign to conventional Western science, including the belief that human beings are composed of and emanate energy fields and that "sickness" results from an imbalance in these fields. It assumes that these energy fields interact and that healthy people can transfer energy to sick people, promoting wellness. In this way, therapeutic touch differs from faith healing or psychic healing, since both of those treatments depend in part on the faith of the person being healed. Therapeutic touch depends entirely on the intent of the healer, who assumes a calm, focused state of concentration. While in this altered state of consciousness, the healer moves his or her hands about four to six inches above the body of the patient. The goal is to detect excess energy, which indicates accumulated tension or illness, and to redistribute that energy, relieving symptoms and promoting health. Thus, therapeutic touch shares ideas with Chinese and Indian medicines, both of which describe a bodily energy that can be rearranged with the help of an external healer.

As foreign as such ideas may sound to us, the notion that touch can heal has long standing in Western culture. At the very least, touching seems to be a near-universal act of

Touch is a near-universal act of human sharing. In one recent experiment, premature babies who were frequently touched gained weight faster than those who were not.

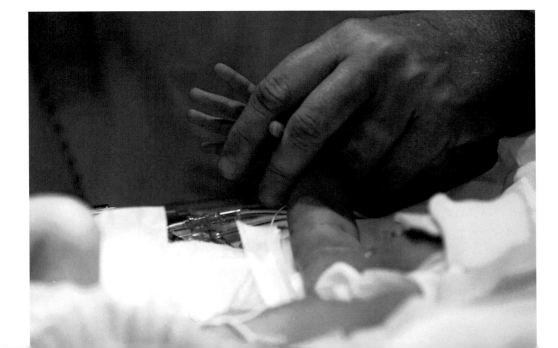

human sharing. A pat on the back or a warm hug lets others know that we share their discomfort and want to help. Fifteen thousand-year-old cave paintings in the Pyrenees include images of caring touch. The Old and New Testaments describe more formal healings through the "laying-on-of-hands," and church records through the Middle Ages endorsed such healings.

Western researchers—many of them nurses—are now demonstrating that therapeutic touch can heal, although we are not exactly sure how. In controlled studies therapeutic touch has been found to encourage relaxation, decrease postoperative pain, relieve headache, and raise the hemoglobin level in the blood. One study involved sixty heart patients at St. Vincent's Medical Center in New York. Each patient received the same therapeutic touch treatment, with one crucial difference. Half the nurses were taught to center themselves calmly and to concentrate on the healing while passing their hands over the patient. The other half were told simply to pass their hands over the patient while mentally counting backward from one hundred by sevens. The researcher, Dr. Janet Quinn, videotaped the sessions and showed them to independent evaluators, who were unable to tell which nurses were concentrating on healing and which were not. Apparently, the *patients* could tell. Anxiety levels were tested before and after each treatment, and the patients who'd received the therapeutic touch showed an average decrease in anxiety of 17 percent. Patients whose nurses were not concentrating on the treatments showed no such change.

One of the lessons of research into therapeutic touch is that we are all potential healers. Healing is not reserved for "sensitives" or "psychics." It is the intent to heal that is all-important. The power of therapeutic touch resides in the special attitude of the healer. By developing a healing attitude, we all may be able to develop that healing touch.

possibly be trained to create a state of internal relaxation, eliminating the driving need to drink. Researchers before him had noticed that the brains of alcoholics seemed dominated by beta waves (associated with thought) and had noticeably fewer alpha and theta waves (associated with relaxation, imagery, and daydreaming). The technique Peniston employed would be largely familiar to anyone who has done a relaxation or imagery exercise, but with this difference: His subjects—patients at Veterans Administration Hospital in Fort Lyon, Colorado—were wired to computers that measured their brain waves and fed them back as a set of tones in a pair of earphones. By working to increase the tones associated with alpha and theta waves, the subjects could measure the success of their relaxation efforts.

Peniston's first step in teaching his subjects to relax was to show them how to raise the temperature of their fingers, which is linked to an increase in theta wave production. They then sat in a darkened, soundproof room for fifteen thirty-minute training sessions. Peniston asked the men to close their eyes and to visualize themselves not drinking, or rejecting a drink. "Imagine your alpha rhythms increasing," he told them. "Sink down into a state of reverie, with your mind quiet and alert and your body calm." With each session the men gradually were able to increase the calming and imagery-associated activity of their brains. Moreover, the alcoholics felt better after the training and showed markedly reduced levels of depression on a standardized test. Most remarkable, thirteen months after the training was over, only two of the ten men had suffered an alcoholic relapse, significantly fewer than in the control group, in which alcoholics received only standard drug and group therapy treatments.

No one is certain why the alcoholics receiving the biofeedback training did so well, since alcoholism is a complex and little-understood disease. What Peniston discovered, however, was that relaxation through brain-wave training seemed to prevent an increase in the levels of the brain chemical beta-endorphin in the blood of his subjects. Beta-endorphin increases with stress and decreases under conditions of relaxation and may be one of many chemicals whose rising and falling levels affect how we feel and perhaps whether we feel the need to take a drink.

One lesson of the biofeedback revolution is that medical technology does not always have to be intrusive. We usually think of new medical machines and innovations as treating us, rather than as helping us find new ways to treat ourselves. The implications of biofeedback and other such techniques are limited only by our level of knowledge, maintains Dr. Brucker of Jackson Hospital. One day, biofeedback technology may enable us to identify and use individual brain cells, which, in turn, may allow us to control the wide array of internal chemical messengers that seem to play such an important role in both health and disease. "As we learn more about the brain," Brucker has said, "and as we develop more advanced microprocessor technology, it may be possible to alter many physiological responses now thought to be beyond human control."

The Magic of the Group

The growing evidence that health is directly related to social support and connectedness to others has led, in recent years, to the establishment of therapy groups for people with everything from drug dependency to cancer. Most such groups serve multiple purposes for their participants. In addition to sharing information about health and disease, members often reinforce behavioral change, by offering praise, understanding, and encouragement. Alcoholics Anonymous, one of the earliest and most successful health-oriented groups, was founded in part in recognition of the value of mutual support. Groups also help members change the way they think about themselves and their situations by discouraging defeatist, self-absorbed, pessimistic thinking and helping members achieve a better perspective on health and disease. In some groups, participants learn to use specific healing tools—such as meditation or imagery—or take on special projects. An AIDS support group in Los Angeles, for example, produced a play about living with AIDS.

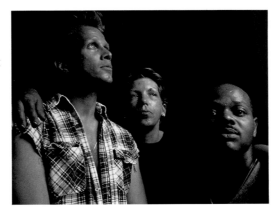

The primary benefit of groups may be that they allow people to share feelings and emotions, reducing social isolation and increasing the sense of connectedness that research has so clearly tied to health. In a highly mobile, individualistic society such as ours, groups often offer a way of establishing honest and open bonds with others. Such support may lift depression and its inhibition of immune function. Psychologists understand the emotional benefits of sharing feelings in a protected environment. As research blurs the line between mind and body, we should not be surprised that groups can help people achieve physical changes as well.

One tantalizing piece of evidence of the power of groups emerged in 1989 with the publication of a study by Dr. David Spiegel of Stanford University. Spiegel divided into two matched groups patients with breast cancer that had spread to other parts of their bodies. Both groups received standard chemotherapy and radiation treatments, but only one group met regularly for peer support, psychotherapy, and self-hypnosis. Ten years later, members of that peer-support group had lived an average of twice as long as the members of the control group: thirty-six months versus eighteen months. Every member of the control group had died, but three of the fifty women in the group that received psychotherapy were still alive.

One reason that group support and sharing may be good for health is that disclosing one's traumatic thoughts and feelings seems to decrease stress and build immunity. To test this, scientists randomly picked twenty-five healthy college undergraduates at Southern Methodist University and asked them to write about trivial issues for twenty minutes a day, for four days in a row; twenty-five other students were asked to write about traumatic issues. The students assigned to write about traumatic subjects addressed such topics as homesickness, death, problems with parents and members of the opposite sex, loneliness, and serious injury or illness. Students in the other group wrote about such trivial subjects as the shoes they were wearing or a recent social event. The researchers measured the students' immune function and also gained their permission to check how frequently they visited the campus health center. The researchers found that the students who wrote about traumatic issues had not only higher immune responses than the members of the "trivial" group, but also a larger drop in health center visits. Moreover, the students who benefited most were the ones who wrote about the subjects they had never before discussed with anyone.

Cardiologist Dean Ornish has made group support an ongoing part of his treatment program. In 1990, Dr. Ornish and his associates published a study in *Lancet*, Britain's most prestigious medical journal, suggesting that heart disease could be reversed through a comprehensive program of diet, stress reduction, exercise, lifestyle changes, and group support. Heart disease occurs when accumulations of fat clog the arteries that supply the heart with blood. Treatment often focuses on cholesterol-lowering drugs and coronary bypass surgery, during which healthy arteries from elsewhere in the body are transplanted to the heart to create a new blood supply. In balloon angioplasty, a newer treatment, a tiny balloon is guided into a

Support groups offer interpersonal sharing, reducing social isolation and promoting connectedness. Group members also share information about drugs, treatments, and coping strategies and reinforce healthful behavior in one another. The photos on these pages show members of Bailey House, a New York City shelter for people with AIDS. Opposite page: Three of the house "cheerleaders." This page: A resident receives a therapeutic massage from a shelter volunteer.

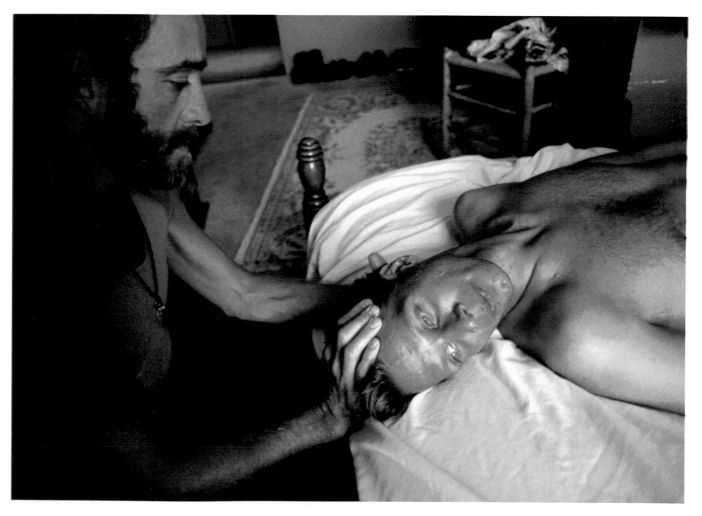

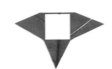

The 2,800 members of the Shanghai Cancer Recovery Club would not be surprised to learn that self-efficacy and taking charge of healing have been shown to improve health. It is as if the club's founders listed all the personal and emotional factors known to promote health—optimism, laughter, love, purpose, spiritual alignment, group support—and set out to help members achieve each one.

A simple encounter with members of the club on one of their many outings makes clear the pride with which they steer this course. Headed south from Shanghai to celebrate the Festival of the Harvest Moon in the lovely city of Hangzhou, club members in uniform white hats hold an impromptu joke fest and sing-along in the aisles of a swaying railway car. Later, they thread the lakes and temples of Hangzhou in a long line, practicing Guo Ling qigong, a form of walking meditation that they believe is saving their lives. They swing their arms in front of them, as if rocking a baby, and breathe in a rhythmic *whoosh, whoosh, whoosh*. Lest anyone wonder who they are, the leader of the line carries a huge red flag bearing the club's name in Chinese. Only two English letters stand out in bold type: CA, for "cancer."

Such public acknowledgment of their cancer would be unusual in most societies. It is especially so in China, where the disease was long misunderstood to be contagious and cancer patients are often ostracized. Nor does China have a tradition of voluntary support or service groups for patients with specific diseases. Partly for this reason, the Shanghai Cancer Recovery Club has attracted a lot of press in China, and similar support groups are beginning to be organized in other Chinese cities.

The club began as a Guo Ling qigong practice group in 1983. Qigong is a three-thousand-year-old meditative discipline that seeks to promote, through exercises and bodily control, the smooth flow of the body's inner energy, or *chi*. A woman named Guo Ling, herself a former cancer patient, modified traditional qigong to emphasize movement and action and especially an increased intake of oxygen during breathing. After Guo Ling began teaching in Shanghai in the 1970s, her method developed a reputation as a cure for cancer.

The theoretical basis of qigong is more widely accepted in China than it would be in the West. China has an ancient tradition of medicine based on the flow of bodily energy, and many Chinese practice tai chi, qigong, and other moving meditations as a kind of health-maintenance tonic. Most cancer patients in China first and primarily receive chemotherapy, radiation, and other Western medical

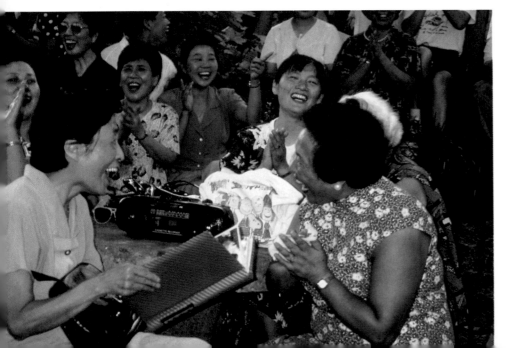

These two pages: The members of the Shanghai Cancer Recovery Club fight cancer with Western medicine, Chinese medicine, a meditation-in-motion called Guo Ling qigong, and a kind of group spiritual therapy—including joke therapy and the promotion of certain long-surviving members to the status of "cancer stars."

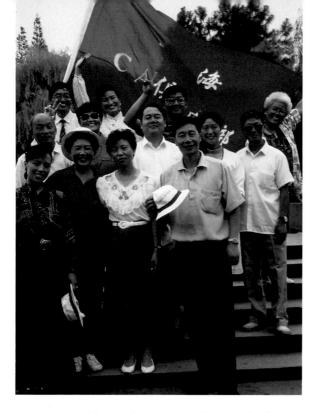

treatments. Many also receive Chinese herbal medicines to balance their *chi* and reduce the side effects of the Western therapies. For patients in the Shanghai Cancer Recovery Club, Guo Ling qigong is one more crucial technique for restoring health.

Wah Nai Zi, a club leader, testifies to the value of Guo Ling qigong. In 1982, when Wah was fifty-two years old, he was rushed to a hospital after losing consciousness because of bleeding due to stomach cancer. As he regained consciousness, Wah overheard a doctor telling his wife to prepare for the worst. The next day, doctors removed four-fifths of Wah's stomach. The surgery was followed by five series of chemotherapy treatments and five years of Chinese herbal medicines. At the same time, Wah sought out a qigong group, at the urging of his wife. "I was not sure it would work," Wah remembers, "but I thought it wouldn't hurt to try. After three months of consistent practice the qigong exercises began to produce results. I could eat better and sleep better. I have continued practicing ever since."

Wah also teaches qigong at one of the fourteen training programs that the Guo Ling qigong club sponsors in Shanghai. For newly diagnosed cancer patients, the club provides cancer "information desks," which are staffed by cancer survivors of at least five years' standing. The group also spreads its message to cancer patients in area hospitals, where it is not surprising to see patients out of bed gliding around the wards practicing Guo Ling qigong.

The recovery club publishes a newsletter, sponsors lectures on various cancer treatments, and organizes diverse activities, from excursions in the countryside to disco dancing for seniors. The club promotes joke-telling contests and sing-alongs, and it sponsors "birthday" celebrations to commemorate the anniversary of each member's cancer diagnosis. In other ceremonies, it elevates to the status of "cancer star" members who have survived cancer in a particularly dramatic way.

The purpose of all of these activities is to provide a kind of group spiritual therapy, which club members see as the fourth leg supporting recovery, along with Western medicine, Chinese medicine, and qigong. "We always say, if you want to live long, you must improve your life's quality," says Yuan Zheng-ping, another of the club's leaders. "Those patients who join the club understand that cancer does not equal death. Their health is strengthened, they have high spirits, stay in a good mood, sleep well and have good appetites."

According to club leaders, members survive longer and enjoy fuller lives than other Chinese cancer patients. Although these claims have never been studied scientifically, the stories of Wah and other club members fit well with what others — both scientists and nonscientists — are learning about the effect of attitude and mind on disease and health. As such stories accumulate, common themes emerge: the crucial importance of optimism, purpose, laughter, connectedness, ritual practice, meditation and other altered states, and a sense of control and efficacy in the face of disease. The universality of these themes ultimately may be the best evidence of the powerful influence of mind and spirit on health.

clogged artery using an x-ray, then briefly inflated to dilate the artery and restore blood flow.

Dr. Ornish began studying alternative treatments for heart disease after noticing that drugs, surgery, and angioplasty usually offered only temporary relief from symptomatic chest pain and the danger of heart attack. Drugs and surgeries definitely helped some patients, Ornish believed, especially in acute, emergency situations, but he wondered if a balanced program of behavioral and dietary changes might not provide the only real healing of the human heart. The program he proposed included not only a low-fat diet and increased exercise—which most physicians recommend—but also stress reduction and a change in the patients' attitudes and social isolation, which Ornish suspected to be one root of the disease.

Dr. Ornish divided patients with severe heart disease into two matched groups. Members of one group followed standard medical recommendations: They ate a moderately low-fat diet, increased their level of exercise, and didn't smoke. Members of the second group were asked to exercise and not smoke, but they also were placed on a diet

The most common form of heart disease occurs when fatty deposits narrow the coronary arteries that supply blood to the heart muscle. These deposits may be due not only to the amount of fat in the diet, but to hormones and other chemicals released under emotional stress. Recent studies have suggested that deposits can be prevented and can actually be reversed through an intensive program of stress reduction, diet, lifestyle changes, and group support. Such interventions are far cheaper—and, for many patients, at least as effective—as standard surgical treatments for heart disease.

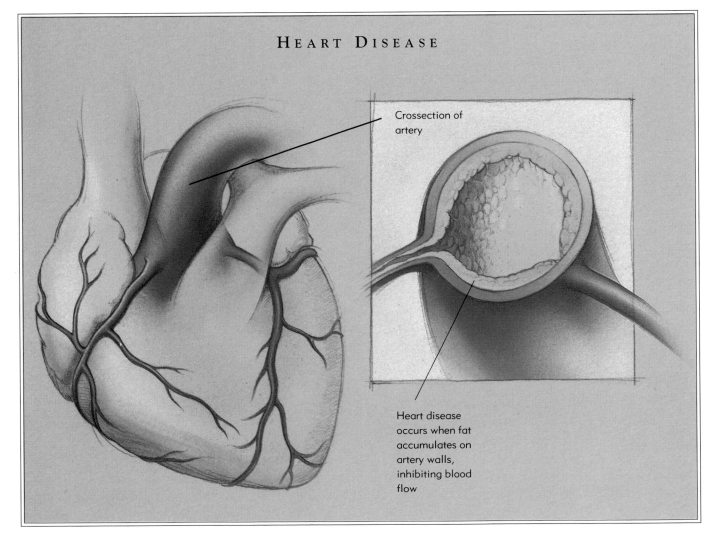

HEART DISEASE

Crossection of artery

Heart disease occurs when fat accumulates on artery walls, inhibiting blood flow

much lower in fat, were taught yoga, meditation, and other relaxation techniques, and met regularly for group support.

In comparing the results from the two groups, Ornish had access to the very latest diagnostic technology. Cardiac angiograms showed that the majority of those patients who followed the standard medical recommendations became measurably worse, whereas 82 percent of the patients who made comprehensive lifestyle changes reduced the average degree of blockage of their arteries. Blockages that had taken a lifetime to accumulate decreased an average of more than 5 percent in only a year. What specifically caused the reversal of heart disease in these patients? Perhaps different things for different patients, Ornish concluded. What was important was that the program as a whole helped most participants begin to reverse their heart disease.

But if there was one portion of the program that seemed to grow in importance over time, it was the group's regular support meetings. Originally, Ornish believed that the meetings would be mostly pep talks, to support and encourage changes in diet, stress management, exercise, and smoking habits. But gradually he realized that the chance to share, to support and gain the support of other people, was one of the most important parts of the treatment program. This recognition, in turn, was based on his growing understanding that heart disease cannot be healed without addressing its root causes. Yes, heart disease is related to stress, to hostility, to diet, to genetic differences—and to having high blood cholesterol, which may result from all of these factors. But at its root, Ornish came to believe, the disease was related to isolation and loneliness—these were the causes of the stress that underlay heart disease, as well as many other emotional and physical woes. Heart disease, Ornish decided, was at least in part a disease of the spirit. Although his patients were all different, Ornish said, they seemed to share a sense of isolation: "From parts of themselves and their own feelings; from other people and a sense of community; and from something spiritual, a sense of being part of something larger than oneself."

In Dr. Ornish's support groups, less time is now spent talking about diet and relaxation, and more time is spent talking about patients' inner lives. "With that often comes an amazing sense of relief and transformation, so that a person doesn't have as much rage and doesn't feel the need to go out and beat people up, or for other people to beat themselves up in various ways, or to engage in destructive behaviors such as alcohol and drugs to kill the pain." Participation in a support group is now a central part of Dr. Ornish's coordinated program to reverse heart disease. "When we can experience that connectedness," Dr. Ornish has said, "it carries over into our work, into our families, into relationships with other people in ways that go far beyond just unclogging arteries. Our hearts begin to open in other ways."

The Power of Taking Charge

In a coastal forest on a sunny summer day near the town of Port Alberni, British Columbia, a dozen or so women sit in a semicircle of folding lawn chairs. The women are Native Canadians—"First Nations People" they are called in Canada—who have gathered from villages up and down the coast to learn how to manage, and help others manage, arthritis. No cures are being offered here beneath the firs, spruce, and cedars—no magic pills. Rather, the women are learning about the biology of arthritis, about relaxation for pain control, about staying mobile through simple exercise, about thinking positively rather than negatively. Most important, they are learning to use this knowledge to take charge of their own healing, to cope with a disease that has no cure. In this way, these women are part of one of the most significant self-healing movements of modern times, a movement based on years of research showing that a sense of personal control can be a powerful force for human healing.

The story of this specific treatment program begins in 1979 with an arthritis self-management course at Stanford University. The goal was simple: to teach patients to cope better with the depression, disability, fear, and pain sometimes associated with the disease. Lessons would focus on the anatomy and physiology of arthritis, on nutrition, on maintaining mobility through exercise, and on reducing stress, pain, and depression through simple relaxation techniques.

At Stanford Children's Hospital, in California, thirteen-year-old girl Kristy Poindexter sits before an elaborate electronic keyboard. Beside her is Joan Avanzino, a music therapist who is helping Kristy deal with the pain and frequent hospitalizations resulting from her chronically inflamed intestines. Kristy pushes keys and spins dials, listening for a specific combination of sounds. She is translating into music a story she has created— a collection of images really, involving a crashed spaceship, a tropical island, a meeting with friendly natives, a storm, and finally a wedding celebration. When she is done, she will have a permanent tape of her own music. The hope is that listening to the tape will induce relaxation and healing.

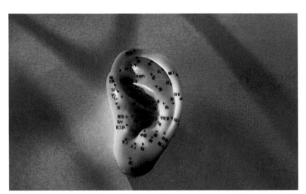

The link between music and health is ancient and elemental. From the earliest thump of our mother's heart to the last whisper of our own expiring breath, our lives are circumscribed by natural rhythms and melodies. We are tied to the Earth by the music of wind-ruffled leaves or the lap of the sea on the shore. Human-made music can delight us, annoy us, enliven us, or soothe us. It touches our emotions and our intelligence and can move us to do great things.

Studies have found that the chills, tingles, and goose bumps we feel while listening to music may be due in part to the release of endorphins, the morphinelike chemicals in the brain. Our bodies respond so acutely to music that it influences heart rate, breathing, and contractions of the stomach. It is probably no accident that most music in Western culture contains between seventy and eighty beats per minute, the approximate rate of the human heart.

In most cultures throughout history, music, dance, rhythmic drumming, and chanting have been essential parts of healing rituals. Modern research bears out the connection between music and healing. In one study, the heart rate and blood pressure of patients went down when quiet music was piped into their hospital coronary care units. At the same time, the patients showed greater tolerance for pain and less anxiety and depression. Similarly, listening to music before, during, or after surgery has been shown to promote various beneficial effects—from alleviating anxiety to reducing the need for sedation by half. When researchers played Brahms's "Lullaby" to premature infants, these babies gained weight faster and went home from the hospital sooner than babies who did not hear the music. Music may also affect immunity by altering the level of stress chemicals in the blood. An experiment at Rainbow Babies and Childrens Hospital found that a single thirty-minute music therapy session could increase the level of salivary IgA, an immunoglobulin that protects against respiratory infections.

Music therapy is particularly beneficial to the elderly. Coupled with gentle exercise, listening to music relieves pain and promotes motion in a way that exercise alone cannot do. Neurologist Oliver Sacks recounts how some patients with parkinsonism and other brain diseases respond to music in truly extraordinary ways: "One sees parkinsonian patients unable to walk, but able to dance perfectly well, or patients almost unable to talk, who are able to sing perfectly well." Sacks describes one patient who sat virutally motionless except when she sat down at the piano, where she at once develped fluidity and grace. Listening to Chopin—her favorite composer—would cause an increase in her measurable brain activity from comalike slowness to near-normal levels.

The legendary power of music to heal may relate to the way it is processed in the brain. Music often bypasses the higher, thinking centers of the brain and appeals directly to the deeper levels—like a mantra used in meditation or an image conjured in the mind. In this sense, music is made up of images received by the ear. Music can grab the brain's attention, creating a special state of consciousness during which easygoing, repetitive melodies may lead to relaxation, while upbeat tunes may leave us feeling invigorated and alive. This state in which music holds the brain's attention may explain why listening to music can block pain. Pain and tension are intimately connected; pain leads to tension, which leads to pain. Soothing music can short-circuit this pain cycle, which is why some dentists use Beethoven or Bach as a kind of aural anesthesia.

Kristy Poindexter is also using music to break the pain and tension cycle. In composing her own work, however, she is pushing the healing power of music to another level. Rather than responding to images in other peoples' music, Kristy is creating her own musical images, drawing on the issues in her own life, including her battle with disease. As Kristy listens to the music, she will experience these images again. The spaceship will crash, the storm will come, just as there have been crashes and storms in Kristy's own life. In the music, however, the friendly natives arrive, and the music ends with a wedding celebration. "When Kristy listens to the tape it will help her process these images again and again," therapist Joan Avanzino says. And in reliving these images while in a relaxed state of consciousness, Kristy may more easily resolve issues subconsciously than she could by "thinking them through." Music can help a person integrate experiences and emotions, Avanzino says: "Music can be very healing in terms of making a person whole."

This approach was a success by almost any standards. Participants experienced less pain, increased their knowledge of arthritis, and were more likely to exercise and participate in other self-management activities than before the course. But the findings were also puzzling. The patients experiencing the greatest pain reduction—those for whom the program seemed to provide the greatest benefits—were not those who had learned the most or even those who engaged in the most self-management activities. If knowledge and behavioral changes did not explain the improvement, what did?

The answer began to emerge in the early 1980s, at a Christmas party in a Stanford home, where Dr. Halsted Holman, an immunologist with the program, encountered Dr. Albert Bandura, a psychologist who was interested in the way people change when they confront and master challenges. Holman told Bandura about the puzzling research findings. Bandura responded that he had a hunch what the answer might be.

Dr. Bandura had done pioneering work with phobias, measuring changes in bodily stress chemicals and immune function in people confronting overwhelming fear. From this work, it had become clear that a sense of mastery—what Bandura called "self-efficacy"—could have far-reaching and positive effects on human psychology and physiology. For one experiment, Bandura had recruited people who were terrified of snakes. The group included people who could not cross open fields or go hiking or camping for fear they would encounter a snake, plumbers who could not bring themselves to work under houses, geologists who avoided field work, and telephone repairmen who could not get to some telephone poles. One woman couldn't bring herself to sit on the toilet of her San Francisco home after reading that a snake had escaped into the Santa Barbara sewer system, more than three hundred miles away.

Bandura assessed his subjects' "perceived self-efficacy" about snakes by asking them a series of questions. Could the subject enter a room with a snake? Put a hand on a snake's cage? Handle a snake? Let the snake touch the subject's face? Researchers also took baseline measurements of the subjects' heart rate, immune function, and cortisol, a stress chemical.

Then, in the next stage of the experiment, supported and guided by a researcher, subjects gradually got closer and closer to a snake, periodically answering the questions again about how close they thought they could get to a snake.

The key to Bandura's phobia treatment is breaking the task down into easily mastered steps. Not surprisingly, as subjects were able to get closer to the snake, their perceived ability to cope with it changed. Measurements showed that immune function—rather than remaining the same, or even decreasing, under the stress of the test—actually increased at exactly the point when the subjects made the greatest change in self-efficacy, at exactly the point they said to themselves, "I can do this."

A similar process might be at work with the arthritis subjects, Bandura suggested to Holman. With this in mind, the Stanford researchers took another look at the graduates of the arthritis program. Indeed, it did seem that the ones who had improved most had the most positive attitudes and most felt a sense of control over the disease. Those who believed the disease to be unconquerable failed to improve, no matter how much attention they paid to nutrition, exercise, and other self-help techniques. On the basis of this knowledge, the researchers reorganized the program to maximize the sense of self-efficacy. In six two-hour weekly sessions, participants were encouraged to set goals to be pursued in small, easily achievable steps. A little success was deemed more important than great effort, since success builds the positive attitude that relieves the symptoms of the disease. Underlying every lesson of the new program was a single, all-important goal: Participants, in the words of the course

These two pages: The conquering of snake phobias has provided an important model for researchers interested in effects of self-efficacy on health. People who conquer phobias under experimental conditions show increases in immune function at exactly the point they say to themselves, "I can do this."

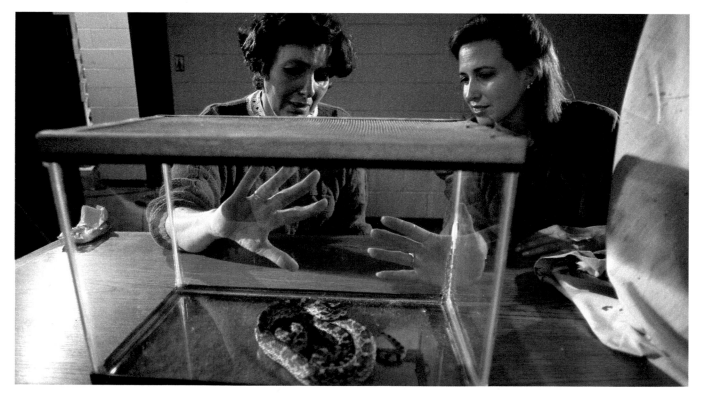

handbook, would "develop more confidence in themselves as caretakers for their bodies."

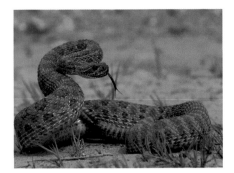

Subsequent research has found that participants in Stanford's arthritis program experience a 20 percent reduction in pain, a 15 percent reduction in depression, a 40 percent reduction in visits to physicians, and a 20 percent increase in social activity. By 1990, the program had trained more than one hundred thousand people, and has been given in Australia, New Zealand, and Canada, where The Arthritis Society offers classes to, among many others, the First Nations People of the British Columbia coast. Self-efficacy has also been linked to success in the treatment of other health problems. The way a person feels about being able to accomplish a task has been found to be important in pain management, heart disease rehabilitation programs, the treatment of eating disorders, and efforts to quit smoking. At the same time, the notion has emerged that pushing through fear and adversity to a sense of self-efficacy can encourage personal growth and health in most people. This notion is behind such outdoor adventure programs as Outward Bound, in which people spend several days to several weeks pursuing daring tasks that test their personal limits. The surge of exhilaration that accompanies climbing a thirty-foot-high tottering pole, for example, or crossing a swaying rope bridge, is a complex mind-body experience from which a new sense of control, accomplishment, and possibility can emerge—which may in turn lead to improved health and balance.

In their research on self-efficacy, the Stanford group has expanded its explorations to include chronic diseases other than arthritis. Chronic diseases—the most common diseases in the developed world—are those for which medicine offers treatments but few cures, including lung and heart conditions, strokes, degenerative bone and joint diseases, and certain cancers and HIV infection. Chronic diseases must be lived with for years, and most of us will get one or more of them if we live long enough. The knowledge that self-efficacy, the belief that we have power over a disease, can be a force in decreasing symptoms and disability could be important news to us all. If the improvements in arthritis patients could be duplicated in patients with other chronic diseases, society would save billions of dollars each year in reduced doctor visits alone. The Stanford researchers already have early indications that patients with chronic lung disease, heart disease, and stroke benefit from courses designed to help them take charge of their disease rather than allowing the disease to take charge of them. This, then, is the bonus benefit of any of the treatments evolving from the new mind-body research. Relaxation and visualization exercises, biofeedback, and group support may all contribute to a sense of control and self-efficacy in the face of disability or disease. Recognition of this benefit is overdue, according to registered nurse Kate Lorig, who coordinates the Stanford program: "The power of people doing things for themselves is very strong medicine, and it has been underrated for a long time."

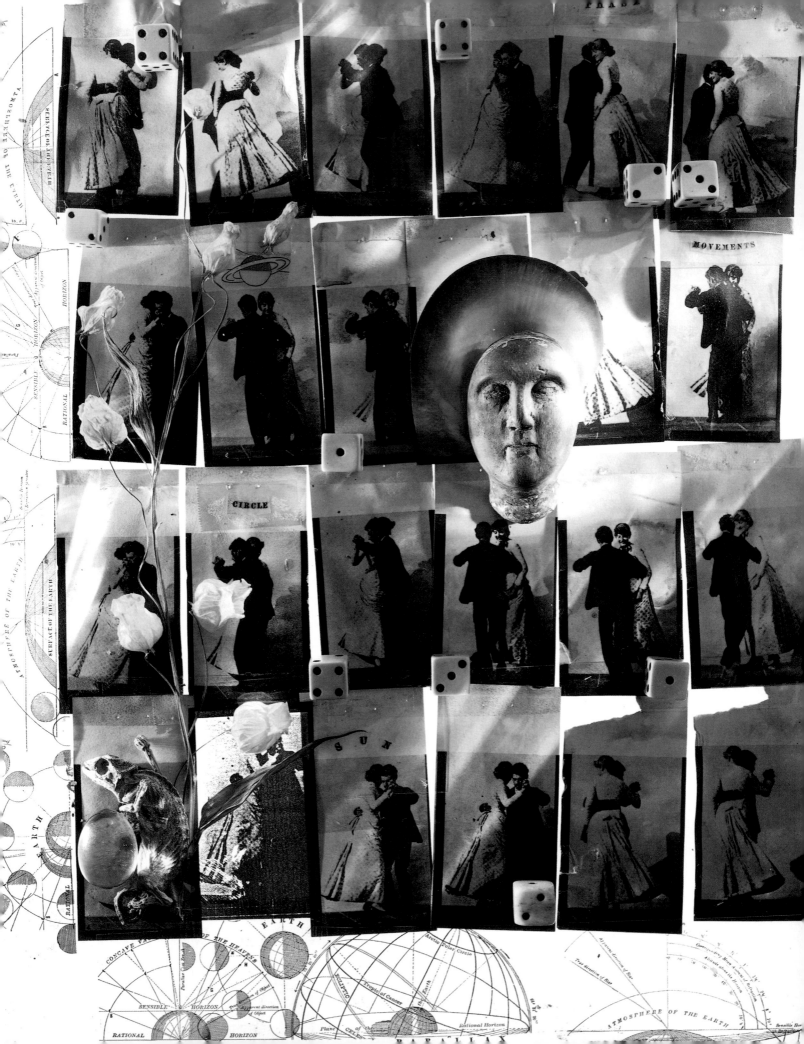

CHAPTER SIX

LIVING AS HEALING

HEALTH, SPIRIT, AND SOCIETY

HEALTH THROUGH THE LIFESPAN

HE WESTERN MEDICAL TRADITION espouses the cookbook approach to health. The standard "recipe" for a healthy life includes recommendations to eat your carrots and broccoli, get plenty of sleep and exercise, avoid known health hazards, and take your medicine when you get sick. But the mind-body conception of health now being rediscovered in our culture suggests the shallowness of cookbook living. The attitudes, values, and personality traits now being linked to health are not so much ingredients in a recipe as they are themes in a biography. They are rooted in genetic inheritance and our upbringing and are deeply affected by the values of the culture in which we live. To take them seriously is to create a whole new view of healing. According to this model, human health depends on a constant interplay between the individual, family, and society. And the ability to heal—physically, emotionally, spiritually—is deeply affected by life events. How we meet life's changing challenges determines not only our physical and mental health, but whether we are able to develop a healing approach to life.

Two questions resonate throughout this final chapter: How do mind-body influences develop through the 7,

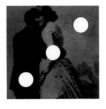

> *"I feel certain that there will come a day when physiologists, poets and philosophers will all speak the same language."*
>
> —CLAUDE BERNARD, FRENCH PHYSIOLOGIST (1813–78)

or 77, or 107 years of life? And how can we create a society—and particularly a medical system—in which the dominant values and attitudes encourage health for all citizens at every stage of life?

The Healing Infant

Suspended in a warm sack of sterile amniotic fluid within its mother's abdomen, the human fetus is nurtured and protected as it never will be again. Temperature is steady. Nutrition and oxygen arrive through the umbilical cord and placenta, along with immunoglobulins to fend off infection, should microorganisms invade the amniotic sack. Then, over a period of several hours, everything changes. Where there was fluid, there is suddenly air, along with the overpowering need to breathe. And soon there is hunger and an instinctive quest for mother's breast. The world surrounding the newborn swarms with microorganisms, which its immature immune system must defend against.

Not that the baby is unprepared. Soon after fertilization, structures and systems begin to form that will regulate the organism's health for a lifetime. In the first weeks of life, cells destined to become immune cells migrate to the fetus's bone marrow. By the fifth month, the fetus is producing its own immune factors to complement what it receives from its mother, and by birth the infant is producing phagocytes to engulf and devour invading bacteria. Throughout these months, the brain and nervous system are also developing.

We now understand that the immune system and the brain and nervous system mature together and are in constant communication, establishing the elaborate network of electrical and chemical communications that will help regulate health and healing for a lifetime. They will continue to develop and change, in part according to a blueprint coded in the genes, and in part because of interaction with physical, social, psychological, and spiritual influences from the environment.

During the last few decades we have learned of many outside influences that can threaten the health of the developing fetus. Cigarette smoking, alcohol consumption, and drug use during pregnancy have been linked to low birth weight or fetal damage, and it is now suspected that a wide range of environmental toxins may cross the placenta to the developing fetus. Less attention has been paid to the health consequences of emotional influences on the fetus and newborn, partly because of a lingering belief that the fetus and infant are not fully conscious and cannot experience emotions, draw conclusions, and attach meaning to experience.

For a long time, scientists believed that because the newborn's motor systems were uncoordinated and underdeveloped at birth, its emotional systems also were uncoordinated and undeveloped. It is gradually becoming clear, however, that fetal and infant experiences not only are recorded but often are remembered, which is important for the development of attachment between the infant and its adult caretakers. This attachment is the infant's first experience in forging the connectedness with other humans that is so closely associated with health. Assuming there is nurturance and dependability in these early relationships, the maturing individual will probably develop ever-widening connections to family, friends, community, and the world.

To an extent, a connection has always existed between the new individual and other human beings, since a developing embryo cannot live without nourishment and support from the mother. Awareness of the connection may come later. A sense of touch begins in the seventh week of the fetus's development, taste blossoms at about fourteen weeks, and hearing is established at eighteen weeks, opening up a prime channel of communication. Fetuses spend many months listening to various rumblings in the mother's gut, the whooshing of blood through veins and arteries, and the rhythmic thump of the mother's heart—which may account in part for the healing agency of rhythm and music for many people later in life. The fetus hears voices as well—particularly and most consistently its mother's voice. Research has shown that a newborn infant already recognizes its mother's voice and prefers it to less familiar voices. Babies tested on a special sucking apparatus at one to three days old are more likely to suck during a story their mother read to them before birth than during a story they've never heard. Similarly, babies show a preference for a melody they heard while in the womb over other melodies.

There is reason to believe that a fetus also may share its mother's stress. In one study the activity of fetuses whose mothers were awaiting routine ultrasound were compared with the activity of those awaiting ultrasound and amniocentesis, in which a needle is introduced through the abdomen and into the amniotic sack for genetic testing. The fetuses of the mothers awaiting amniocentesis were significantly more active, perhaps because they sensed the mothers were anxious. In southern Italy, fetuses who went through an earthquake showed a noticeable increase in activity in ultrasound imaging as much as eight hours later. Other studies have found that pregnant women who are chronically depressed bear significantly more hyperactive babies, and that fetuses become more active when their mothers are shown a frightening video.

After birth, other mechanisms strengthen the mother-infant attachment. The newborn's eyes focus most efficiently at the distance between the mother's

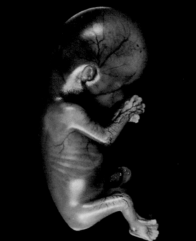

A human fetus is shown (above) at about eighteen weeks old. Even before birth, physical and emotional indluences are at work that may mold health for a lifetime.

breast and face, which the infant quickly learns to recognize. Feeding at the breast of its mother or in the arms of a caretaker, the baby comes to associate physical nurturance with emotional attachment. This attachment is as important to the larger health of the organism as are the nutrients and immune substances in the mother's milk.

It is not crucial that the mother-infant bonding take place immediately after birth. Research has shown that the bond can develop successfully hours or days later—if a mother is recovering after a Cesarean section, for example—or even weeks or months later, as often happens after an adoption. What is important is that the infant establish human contact early and often, that its needs are dependably met, and that it develops a nurturing relationship with its caretakers that expands over time to a trusting connectedness to others. In forming this early attachment, the infant learns to trust the caretaker and feel that the world is a dependable place. Research at the University of Minnesota's Preschool Project has shown that infants who do not establish these early connections face accumulating problems with adjustment by the time they enter preschool. Teachers of such children consistently rate them lower on positive emotions, higher on negative emotions, less emotionally healthy, more dependent on others, and less popular with their peers than classmates who have more secure attachments.

In his landmark 1963 book, *Childhood and Society*, psychiatrist Erik Erikson called the early development of trust the primary task of infant life. All subsequent human development is laid upon this foundation, Erikson believed. He was focusing primarily on emotional health, but there is ample evidence that physical problems also flow from the absence of trusting attachment in the early years. "Failure-to-thrive syndrome" is a condition of infants in which they fail to gain weight, or even die, apparently

THE MEDICALIZATION OF BIRTH

Nothing underscores the advantages and drawbacks of Western technological medicine so acutely as its impact on childbirth. Until a hundred years ago, childbirth was not the province of medicine. Birth was seen as a natural and normal event—although not entirely without difficulty or risk—and most babies were born at home with the help of experienced women attendants or professional midwives. As technological medicine gained influence in the early decades of this century, women went to hospitals to give birth, and midwives gave way to doctors. In the process, birth was transformed from a natural event to a medical procedure and pregnancy was treated as a pathological condition. By the 1960s, delivering a baby in America had acquired all the trappings of high-tech medicine, including fetal monitors, specialized drugs, and a growing tendency among attending doctors to intervene in the birth process at the least sign of fetal distress. A certain percentage of all births carry a life-threatening risk for mother, baby, or both, and no doubt this technology has saved many lives. But the intrusion of technological medicine into birth also has damaged health—especially when health is defined in the larger sense of wholeness.

When the technological model of medicine was most in vogue, the birthing process was totally under the control of obstetricians, most of them men. Women were separated from their husbands and the female care givers who had traditionally supported women in childbirth. The expectant woman was seen as a patient. In this way, the woman was stripped of responsibility for her condition, decreasing her feelings of control and self-efficacy in the face of the pregnancy and birth. Gradually, the technology had taken control of the birth process. For example, when a doctor learned from a fetal monitor that a fetus might be having a problem, he often felt he had to intervene, even though the problem—assuming there was one—might have resolved on its own. This tendency increased because of the threat of lawsuits, in which a doctor could be found negligent for not acting at the slightest suggestion of danger. Most often the intervention took the form of a Cesarean delivery. Today, nearly a quarter of all births in the United States are by Cesarean section, up from only 5 percent in the 1960s.

There is no evidence that these technologies improved infant survival overall. Between 1950 and 1990, the United States dropped from fifth to twenty-first worldwide in the percentage of babies who survived the first year of life. In fact, the countries with the lowest infant mortality rates seem to be those that rely less on obstetricians and more on trained midwives.

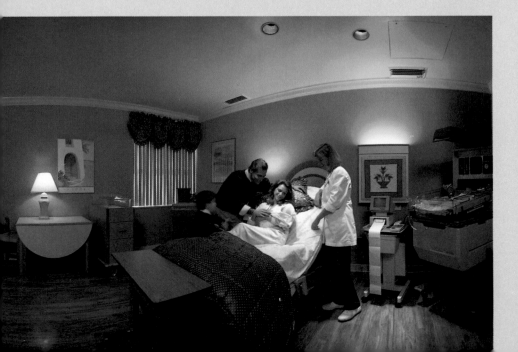

In the middle decades of this century, most American women gave birth in sterile hospital delivery rooms far from the love and support of family and friends. The growing recognition that most births do not need intensive medical supervision has led to the development of homelike hospital birthing rooms (left). Opposite page: Other women with uncomplicated pregnancies choose to give birth at home, perhaps with the help of a trained midwife.

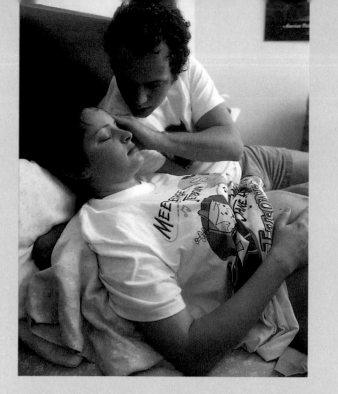

This may be because medical interventions carry their own risks, endangering some babies even as others are saved.

Since the 1970s, there has been a movement to reconfirm birth as a natural process, while at the same time recognizing the value of the life-saving technologies of Western medicine for the women and babies who need them. This movement includes an increase in the percentage of home births, a rediscovery of the role of midwives, and the growth of specialized hospital birthing rooms, where family and friends can stay together during labor and delivery. Across the country, approximately 160 birth centers—most supervised by nurse-midwives—now offer labor and delivery services in a homelike atmosphere. Many are located near hospitals, and all provide medical care if needed. A 1989 study in the *New England Journal of Medicine* found that such birth centers offered a "safe and acceptable alternative" for some women. The goal of such birth practices is to balance wholeness with medicine and old knowledge with new knowledge, to make the best use of technology without letting it dominate the delivery. In this way, the movement to reintroduce more natural birthing is modeling the kinds of changes that need to occur throughout the Western health-care system.

because they do not get enough loving contact. One of the earliest demonstrations of failure to thrive may have occurred as a side effect of an experiment organized by the Holy Roman Emperor Frederick II early in the thirteenth century. Frederick, an amateur scientist, believed that all humans might share an innate language that would emerge naturally if they did not hear another language first. To test this hypothesis, he ordered selected parents to care for their infants' physical needs but not to utter a word in their presence. Reportedly, all the infants died. Something similar happened during World War II, when babies were evacuated from London and kept in large, impersonal nurseries in the countryside. Although they received adequate nourishment, many babies put on weight very slowly, and some lost weight and eventually died.

In addition to being deprived of human attachment, babies raised in this way miss the stimulation that is crucial for growth and health—particularly the health of the developing brain and nervous system. The human brain is immature at birth, and grows, establishes connections, and organizes itself in response to stimulation from the environment. Experiments at the University of California, Berkeley, have shown that shrinkage occurs in the brains of rats raised in cages without toys or other stimulation. Another study has shown how certain kinds of stimulation and experience in babies may affect stress and health later. Researchers at McGill and Stanford universities divided rats into two groups. In one, the rats were removed from their cages and handled for fifteen minutes each day until they were weaned, at about twenty-two days old. The rats in that group showed lower stress hormone responses, not just during infancy but into advanced age.

The stimulation and nurturance of touch have also been associated with physical growth. Scientists at Duke University discovered this by accident when they found stunted growth in rat pups that had been separated from their mothers. This was not due to any difference in nourishment, the scientists discovered, but because the rats' mothers were not licking them. This licking promotes the release of the hormones necessary for growth. Human infants show a similar

In the 1980s, pediatric surgeons began performing operations on human fetuses. After the mother and fetus were anesthetized, the mother's abdomen was opened up along with the amniotic sack, which was drained of fluid. Surgeons then would correct a life-threatening problem in the fetus, before returning the amniotic fluid, closing the mother's abdomen, and allowing the fetus to develop to term. One of the fascinating results of this surgery was the discovery that the babies who had these operations were born with no scars. Had the surgery been performed after birth, massive scarring probably would have occurred. These babies, however, slipped into the world smooth and perfect, as if they'd never known the surgeon's knife. Here was a special kind of healing apparently present only in the developing fetus. Researchers at the University of California, San Francisco, where fetal surgery was developed, have begun studying this capability and have discovered that such healing occurs not only in human fetuses, but in other animal fetuses as well. Unlike wounds created after birth, wounds in fetuses never become inflamed and never form fibrous scar tissue. On the surface and deep into the layers of skin and underlying tissue, the wounded area develops exactly as if it were never wounded at all.

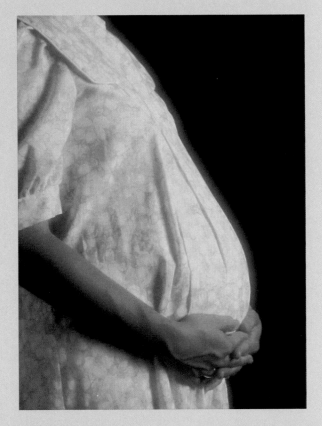

This special ability to heal may be a result of conditions in the womb or knowledge lodged in fetal cells. Researchers have begun delineating how the biochemical events of healing differ in a wounded fetus from those in a wounded adult. They hope one day to apply the secrets of healing in the fetus to wound-healing problems in adults: for example, to alleviate the painful adhesions that sometimes form after surgery. Questions about this special healing abound. Why should the fetus, which, under natural conditions, would rarely suffer wounds, display this unique capability to heal? And why should the way wounds heal change after birth? In that this mode of healing may be carried in our genes, we must wonder what switches off the capability and whether we might be able to learn to switch it on in later life. Answering such questions could be one of the most interesting challenges in the world of healing.

reaction to touch. Because they are born with immature heat-regulating systems, premature babies are usually kept in incubators for warmth, which often isolates them from human contact. At the University of Miami, researchers showed that frequent stroking of premature babies led to weight gains 47 percent higher than in a matched group of infants who were not stroked. The stroked infants were also more active and responsive than the unstroked infants, evidence that the development of their nervous systems was more rapid.

Growing Healthy Children

Receiving the right amount of physical, emotional, and intellectual stimulation remains important to health throughout life. Stress is one form of overstimulation, but understimulation can also be detrimental. For example, scientists are only beginning to recognize the importance of stimulating play to humans and other animals. Many young mammals, birds, and even a few fish and reptiles devote long hours to such seemingly purposeless playful activities as running, somersaulting, bucking, leaping, and spinning. Since such behavior expends valuable energy and often exposes the animals to predators, the return in future health and performance must be great.

One purpose of play is the development of the brain, especially the cerebellum, which coordinates balance, movement, and posture. Researchers have found that in most young animals playfulness peaks at exactly the time when the cerebellum is frenetically establishing connections with the rest of the brain. Although a person may be born with a predisposition to graceful movement and balance, the rigor and stimulation of play helps promote the nervous connections that secure these abilities. But for humans and many other animals, play serves a multitude of other functions. Play helps young animals tame hostile impulses, learn cooperative skills, and rehearse parenting and other adult roles. Children master language in part through play—from the babble games of infants to the intricate invented stories of the school-age child.

Also during childhood, attitudes and values evolve that will be associated with health throughout life.

Through play, school, and home life, children develop pictures of themselves and their relationship to the world. Out of these pictures emerge people characterized by their self-efficacy, optimism, commitment, and trust—or, alternately, their depression, pessimism, and hopelessness. For example, hostility, competitiveness, and other Type A characteristics linked to high stress and heart disease run in families—in part perhaps because these characteristics are genetic, but also because they can be transmitted from parent to child.

In a study led by psychologist Carl Thoresen of Stanford University, children between ten and fourteen years old were divided into groups based on whether they exhibited high or low levels of stress. Each child was assigned a task: to stack blocks one on top of another while wearing a blindfold and with one hand tied behind the back. The child's mother or father was in the room with the child "just to watch," while researchers observed the family behind a one-way mirror. While some parents sat quietly, letting the child tackle the task on his or her own, others fired off a barrage of commands and instructions. One father issued more than 120 commands in eight minutes. Not surprisingly, the children of the most critical, directive parents were the ones who exhibited the most stress.

From this and similar studies, a picture has emerged of the ways parents can pass stress and Type A characteristics onto their kids. In general, parents of Type A children have been found to make more negative and fewer positive comments about their children's performance. They also are more likely to compare their children's performance negatively with that of other children than simply to ask their children to work at their best. The attitude of these parents is not "Do your best and that will be good enough," but "Do your best and it had better be good enough." The result is that parental love becomes conditional, something that must be earned. According to recent research, parents of angry, Type A children are also more likely to use physical and restrictive discipline. Such families offer little support and do not encourage the open expression of feelings. In the movie *The Great Santini*, actor Robert Duvall played such a parent, a hypercritical Air Force fighter

In the Western world, we like to pretend that Western medicine is "scientific," based on physical laws and orderly experimentation, not on cultural preoccupations. In fact, Western medicine has sprouted with great variety, depending on the cultural soil in which it has taken root. Treatments vary widely, and commonly used European remedies may be dismissed as unscientific in the United States. There are even differences in what constitutes an illness: Low blood pressure is treated as an illness in Germany but would entitle an American patient to a lower health insurance rate. In a study by the World Health Organization, researchers provided physicians from different countries with information from death certificates. In many instances the physicians did not agree on the cause of death, even though they reviewed the same certificates.

How you are treated when you feel sick, and even whether you are diagnosed with a disease at all, depend to a large extent on the country in which you were examined. It is only when we understand the links between medicine and culture that we can learn to question medical practices, rather than simply accepting them all as "scientific." Journalist Lynn Payer spent several years researching cultural bias in medicine in England, France, Germany, and the United States. "While medicine benefits from a certain degree of scientific input," Payer concluded, "culture intervenes at every step of the way." Among Payer's observations:

• West Germans are preoccupied with their hearts. In Germany, many patients complaining of common fatigue are diagnosed with Herzinsuffizienz (roughly translated as "weak heart"), a disease with no equivalent in England, France, or the United States. In the German romantic tradition, the heart is viewed not simply as a circulatory device but as the seat of emotion. West Germans consume approximately six times as many heart stimulant drugs per capita as do the French and English but are prescribed half as many antibiotics as other Westerners. This is perhaps the legacy of pioneer German physician Rudolf Virchow, who believed that internal weaknesses, and specifically insufficient blood circulation, were primarily responsible for disease. "If a patient needs an antibiotic," one physician told Payer, "he generally needs to be in the hospital."

• The French also emphasize internal weakness as the cause of disease. This extends from the concept of le terrain (roughly meaning "the soil"), developed at the time of the great French physicians Louis Pasteur and Claude Bernard. According to Payer, "much of French medicine is an attempt to shore up the terrain with tonics, vitamins, drugs and spa treatments. One out of two hundred medical visits in France results in the prescription of a three-week cure at one of the country's specialized spas." And while the Germans may be preoccupied with their hearts, the French have traditionally blamed diseases on their livers. Cris de foie, liver crisis, was at one time a popular diagnosis for everything from headache to impotence.

• English medicine, like American medicine, tends to focus on external causes of disease. Few tonics, vitamins, and spas are prescribed by English physicians, who offer correspondingly more antibiotics to combat bacteria. Otherwise, English physicians are known for their tendency to prescribe fewer drugs, treatments, and surgeries than other Western physicians. Part of the reason is cost: Unlike doctors in other Western countries, British physicians are paid a salary or flat fee to care for each patient, no matter how much work the treatment entails. Certain heart procedures, such as angiography (a computer-assisted study of the heart) and coronary bypass surgery, are six times less common in England than in the United States. In one

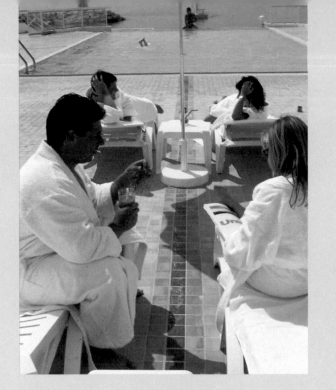

A solarium and relaxation area by an outdoor pool sit on the Mediterranean, and are part of a center that offers people therapy with sea water.

study, British and American doctors were shown identical case histories and tests and asked to evaluate whether patients would benefit from such procedures. After cost issues were set aside, British physicians were still two to three times less likely to regard the procedures as appropriate.

• In American medicine, by contrast, aggressive treatment is the norm. In general, American physicians seem to believe that *some* treatment, *any* treatment, is always better than letting nature take its course. American physicians prescribe more tests than their counterparts in Europe, and they perform more surgeries—including twice the number of hysterectomies and Cesarean sections per capita—as in most European countries. Payer traces this tendency to the American pioneer spirit, the sense that we had to take charge to conquer the frontier. More specifically, she traces it to eighteenth-century American physician Benjamin Rush, who declared the "undue reliance on the power of nature in curing disease" to be one of the primary obstacles to the development of medicine.

pilot whose stress and hostility spilled over into his family life and ultimately erupted in violence against his son.

Fortunately, other parents promote health-building attitudes in their children—such as self-efficacy and an optimistic view of the self. Like the rest of us, children learn these attitudes in part from their own daily accomplishments and triumphs. "Mommy, Mommy, look what I can do!" may be the most commonly heard cry of the young child. How Mommy and Daddy and teachers and other adults respond to a child's efforts over the years can be crucial in developing the attitudes so often associated with good health. Parents can encourage optimism and self-efficacy in their children by modeling these attitudes themselves. They can be consistent and positive and set reasonable goals for success. They can encourage their children to regard failures as individual events and not as part of a pattern of failure. Finally, they can interpret success as consistent with the child's ongoing mastery of the world's challenges.

Toward Adulthood

Achieving health, in all senses of that word, is a cumulative accomplishment. At each stage in our lives we build upon attitudes and coping styles learned in the stages before. At no time is this foundation shaken as much, however, as it is in adolescence. Social connectedness is threatened as relationships are realigned. Optimism, self-efficacy, and self-worth are challenged by new and often complicated tasks. Relationships become intimate, schools and careers get chosen, futures are planned. It is a risky time for health. Accidents, suicide, and homicide are among the leading causes of death in adolescents. And, as they struggle to establish individual identities, adolescents often push the boundaries of healthy behavior. Suddenly, what parents and authority figures say about health becomes less important than the opinions of peers. Health habits are established in these years that may later be hard to break, including smoking and the feel-good fix of drug and alcohol abuse. It is as adolescents that most of us first consider seriously the meaning and purpose of life, as the uncritical idealism of childhood collides with the analytical abilities of the adult. The adolescent learns that there are different standards for human happiness, different philosophies of life.

Our society does not make it easy for adolescents to assume the purposeful and committed adult roles associated with health. A lengthy adolescence, separate from other life stages, is a modern creation to educate the young for increasingly complex adult roles. In the majority of the world's cultures, through most of human history, those roles—as warriors, hunters, gatherers, farmers, caretakers—were clear, and young people knew what was expected of them. Transitions from one life stage to another were viewed as sacred by the culture's religion and often marked by the rituals that anthropologists call rites of passage. Most people in our culture do not have such secure adult roles. Instead, our culture proposes a career track, and in place of consecrated rites of passage, we offer thin, secularized equivalents, such as high school or college graduation. Thus, many adolescents and young adults spend years trying out roles, seeking a life with an appropriate fit. High rates of drug abuse and emotional problems among the young suggest how many of them fail.

As adulthood progresses, some of us are rewarded generously through our relationships and work. Others never manage to develop the hardiness to buffer the stress of work and family. It is during the adult years that anxiety-related diseases become common, and in mid-life, many people experience a period of personal reassessment, prompted by an imbalance between the rewards and stress of life. The pressures of jobs and careers contribute to this feeling of imbalance. Between 1970 and 1991, a full month was added to the working year of the average American, leaving less time for family and leisure pursuits. For some people, this work has meant increasing wealth, but surveys have shown that greater wealth does not necessarily correlate with greater satisfaction. Rising medical expenses and employee absences due to work-related stress have prompted many companies to hire stress-relief experts. At particular risk are workers who cannot exercise any control over steady, unremitting work. One fascinating suggestion that work may be bad for some people's health is that heart attacks occur more often on Mondays than on any other day—and not just on Mondays, but on Monday mornings at about 9:00 A.M., when the workweek begins for most Americans.

Stresses within the family also take their toll. Marital disagreements can temporarily decrease immunity, and long-standing marital rancor may lead to disease and poor health, especially in women. Women are also subject to stress as they try to balance child rearing with careers. One 1990 survey of mental depression in one thousand families found that the most depressed women were those trying to juggle work and child care while receiving little help from their husbands. Among the least depressed women were working women who either had no children or had access to easy, affordable child care and whose husbands helped with the child-rearing responsibilities.

The Importance of Spirit

In many people, the reassessment in mid-life is prompted by more than accumulating dissatisfactions and stress. A sense of emptiness—a lack of purpose, meaning, and coherence in life—is causing their pain. For them, the crisis is spiritual and its resolution central to establishing that wholeness that is the source of true health.

Spirit is difficult to define and impossible to measure. Yet its existence has been unquestioned across the breadth of human societies. Some people describe spirit as a deep sense of belonging and connectedness. Great religions have been founded to pass on the wisdom of spiritual teachers, to create symbols and rituals as aids to worship, to develop spiritual practice and discipline. Religions help many people experience spirit and incorporate spiritual practice into their lives. But religions do not have an exclusive claim on spirit, which is present and experienced everywhere it is sought. Spirit may be experienced directly, especially by people who seek its presence through prayer and meditation, or observed in its influence on human lives. Spirit may be manifest as altruism—selfless service to others— or as love.

Spirit has been pushed to the edges of our culture

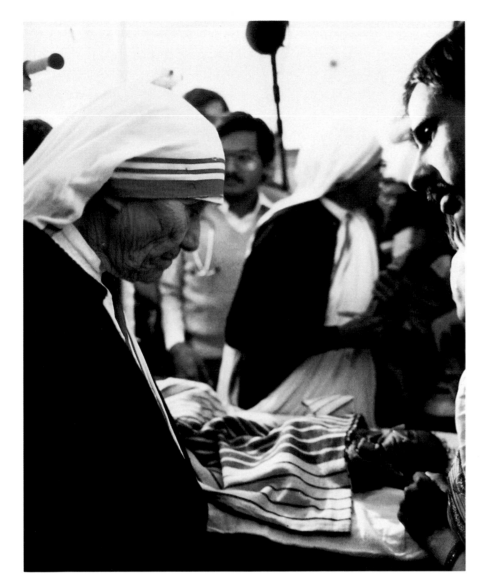

Spirit may be experienced directly or observed in its influence on the lives of others. Love and altruism both reflect the influence of spirit on human lives. Shown here, Mother Teresa of Calcutta, head of the Order of the Missionairies of Charity, ministers to the sick after an industrial gas leak killed 2,500 in Bhopal, India. Mother Teresa won the Nobel Prize for Peace in 1979.

and is not readily acknowledged as a force in everyday life. Our culture is materialistic in a way that transcends its orientation toward money and possessions. Materialism is the philosophical theory that physical matter is the only reality and that everything is ultimately explainable in terms of its physical properties. As discussed in Chapter Two, the Western medical system is founded on this theory, and, consequently, there is not much room for spirit in our medicine.

That spirit cannot be measured makes it hard to "prove" spiritual influences on physical health. Some of the strongest suggestive evidence comes from inexplicable healings such as those at Lourdes (described in Chapter One) and from people who have undergone spontaneous remission from cancer, many of whom report the kind of profound life change associated with spiritual awakening. The association between healing and spirit has also been demonstrated by the success of Alcoholics Anonymous and similar self-help groups. Such groups urge people to seek help from a higher power in taking control of health-

WATER, FIRE, AND THE HEALING SPIRIT

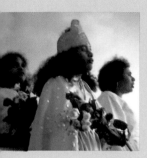

Healing is associated with spirit and spiritual concerns in cultures worldwide. On December 6, a little after six in the morning, a "Umbandista," a follower of the Umbanda faith, walks toward the sea in Praia Grande, on the coast of Brazil, and launches a little boat decked with flowers. Slowly, others from different temple groups join her and launch their boats. Later, some of these faithful will be baptized in every seventh wave. But this sunrise ceremony is not like a Christian baptism—there is no "original sin" to be washed away. Instead, it is regarded as part of a transaction: You cast flowers as offerings upon the waves, and in turn the ocean cleanses and heals you. Some people also carry little coffins, which contain symbols of the negative things they want to cast away and ask the sea to take.

For three days each year, in the summer of Brazil, tens off thousands of followers of the Umbanda faith come to to Praia Grande to participate in the Festival of Iemanja, to worship Iemanja, the goddess of the sea. Many spend the night on the beach in preparation for the ceremony—dancing, playing drums, and going into a trance that lasts until dawn. Healing is at the heart of this ceremony and of the Umbanda faith.

Every weekend, healing ceremonies take place in Umbanda temples, and mediums take on the personalities of spirits and literally "blow away" harmful influences from those people they heal. Appealing to people from every background—rich, poor, Indians, Africans,

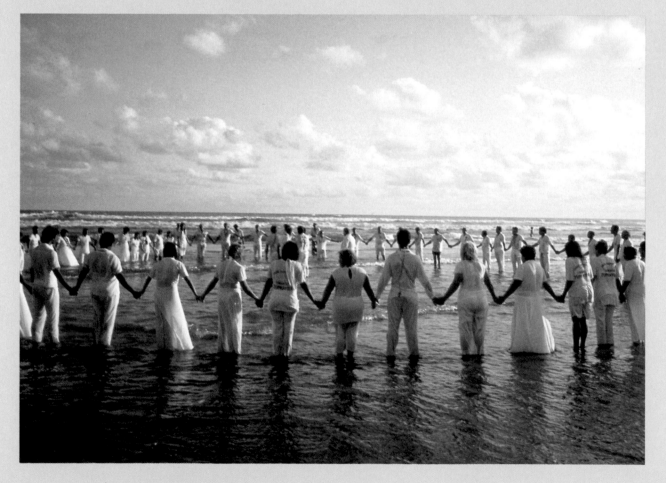

Europeans—the Umbanda religion is the fastest-growing faith the country.

Halfway around the world, members of a Christian sect called the Apostolics also gather regularly to court the healing spirit. Once a year in the remote desert lands of Zimbabwe, they celebrate Passover in a ten-day ceremony. Founded seventy years ago, the Apostolics reject Western medicine and do their best to prevent their children from being inoculated. They believe that the Lord chooses who will survive. The Apostolics gather for the ceremony in the desert for the absolution and the curing of diseases. They believe the Holy Ghost comes among them and heals the body and spirit of those who are pure. Healers wander among the crowds and "cast out" evil spirits.

By the last day of the celebration, men and women have begun to testify, and everyone prays and sings. A giant fire is built on this last evening, and the Apostolics circle it. They believe that God is in the midst of the fire, and as they circle it, they confess their sins, ready to begin the next day cleansed in mind, body, and spirit.

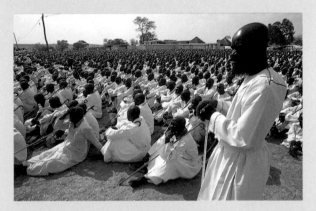

Opposite page: Followers of the Umbanda faith gather at the sea for three days each year to be cleansed and healed by the sea. This page: Once a year, Apostolics gather in the desert for a ten-day ceremony for the absolution of their sins and for their diseases to be cured.

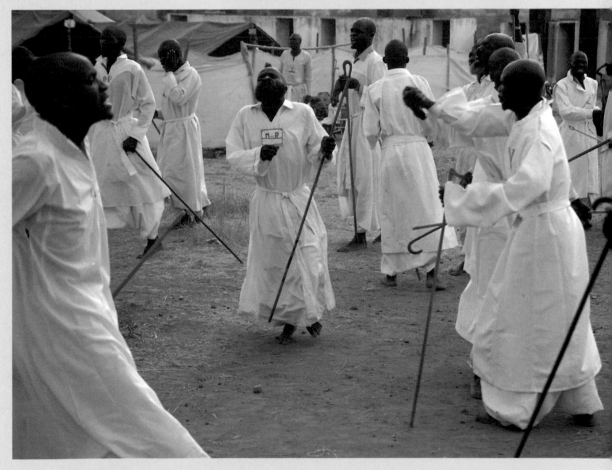

destructive behaviors. The willingness to assume responsibility for one's behavior while at the same time enlisting the influence of spirit can be a powerful force for health.

Sometimes it is possible to measure the influence of spiritual qualities, such as love, altruism, and caring, on health. Harvard psychologist David McClelland showed students a film about Mother Teresa, who won a Nobel Prize for Peace, and her work with Calcutta's poor. All the students, even those who claimed Mother Teresa was a fake, showed an increased secretion of salivary IgA, an immunoglobulin that protects against colds and upper respiratory infections. When the students were shown a film about the Mongol conqueror Attila the Hun, this measure of immunity dropped.

Similarly, certain behaviors sometimes associated with spiritual practice can be measured. In a seventeen-year study in Alameda County, California, church members showed lower mortality than those who were not church members—perhaps due to spiritual factors or because of increased social support or more consistent health habits. And in a study of 2,800 elderly residents of New Haven, Connecticut, those who were involved in a church were less likely to become medically disabled than those who considered church unimportant. Positive mental health—especially the prevention of depression, which has been tied to numerous physical ills—has also been linked to churchgoing. A 1991 review of two hundred studies published in the *Journal of Psychology and Theology* concluded that, in general, churchgoers showed lower suicide rates, lower rates of drug use, lower divorce rates, greater marital happiness, and lower rates of depression.

Several studies have attempted to show the influence of prayer on health and healing. In two studies in the 1960s, researchers were unable to demonstrate any statistically significant improvement in groups of ill patients who were prayed for by others. For a 1988 study, Dr. Randolph Byrd divided 393 patients in a San Francisco coronary care unit into two matched groups. Half the patients were prayed for by an outside group of "born-again" Christians; half were not. Although all the patients knew that the prayers were being said, neither they nor their care givers knew which patients were being prayed for. Byrd then recorded complications that befell the patients during hospitalization, including the need for drugs, treatments, and surgeries. At the end of treatment, 84 percent of the prayed-for group was judged under these criteria to have had a "good" hospital course as opposed to only 73 percent of the control group. The study's results were found to be statistically significant and were published in the *Southern Medical Journal.*

Results such as Byrd's are seized upon by those who have experienced the force of spirit in the world and believe in its power to heal. But why should we measure the efficacy of spirit only by the yardstick of physical improvement? We shouldn't conceive of spirit as we do the magic-bullet drugs and treatments of Western scientific medicine. Byrd's study, for example, did not attempt to measure other, more generally accepted effects of spirit: whether there was a change in the patients' perspectives regarding illness or mortality, or whether they experienced some new insight or found some greater peace.

Toward Healthy Aging

Health becomes an increasing concern as people age. Our bodies begin to let us down. Aches and pains accumulate, and for many, chronic disease sets in. Yet some older people describe this as a time of great peace and purpose. They are less bombarded by life's busyness, and they have more time to concentrate on those things that give them the most satisfaction and meaning. One of the challenges of old age is to maintain this larger sense of wholeness even as physical health may fade.

Many societies venerate the elderly and value their knowledge. Older people help care for the young or tend the home. They help generate a grander vision for the family and the community. The longer a person lives, the more he or she is assumed to have learned. This is especially true of spiritual knowledge, which must be experienced and accumulated over time. In our individualistic culture, however, wisdom held in trust for the community is given little value. As materialists, we too often value people on the basis of their chief material property, their bodies. By this standard, young is better than old, strong is better than weak, attractive is better than ugly, and healthy is better than sick. We are a culture that exalts youth, and it is this prejudice that has brought us the tummy tuck, the facelift, and our preoccupation with appearance. In our capitalist economic system, which values people according to their ability to spend and produce, it is easy to see how self-worth and self-efficacy may suffer as people age.

Other forces work against health and wholeness in the aging. In a society as highly mobile as ours, connectedness is threatened as families grow up and move away, or friends relocate. Too often, older people lose a sense of control over their lives in the face of these changes, sickness, or economic problems. Commitment and purpose may be lost, especially after retirement, since so many of us define our societal value on the basis of jobs and careers. Such losses can affect physical health.

The immune system functions less effectively in the aging years, and the health-controlling brain, nervous system, and hormonal system also decline. This decline is not the same for everyone, however. People age at different rates, in part because of their genetic blueprints, but also because of their nutrition, living conditions, attitudes, and emotional states. As we age, a cycle can develop in which failing health leads to feelings of powerlessness, purposelessness, lack of control, and depression,

History is full of people who remain vital into advanced old age. Psychologists believe that the one key to a productive old age may be a meaningful involvement that keeps an older person oriented toward the future.

Shown here is renowned cellist, pianist, composer, and conductor Pablo Casals conducting the Marlboro, Vermont, festival orchestra in 1971. Casals made music until he died in 1973, at the age of ninety-seven.

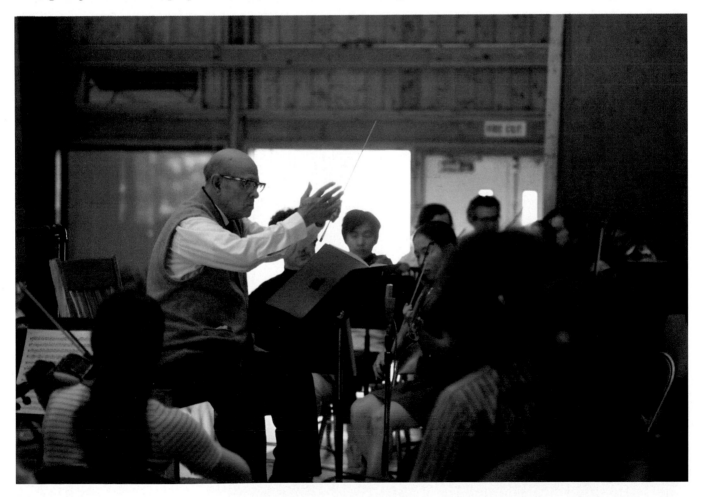

which contribute to failing health. The people who seem to remain the healthiest the longest seem to be those who remain fully engaged in life. Is it any wonder that many of us fear retirement?

Dr. George Solomon, who pioneered PNI research on arthritis patients in the 1960s, has studied the psychological characteristics of the "healthy elderly," people who remain active in mind and body, even at a hundred years old. Solomon became interested in these people while studying long-term survivors of AIDS and began to wonder whether the same characteristics might be found in both groups. He decided they were. "One of these characteristics is an orientation toward the future," Solomon said. "I interviewed one ninety-three-year-old who wanted to buy a new car and was concerned about how well it would hold up. These people are also independent, self-reliant and meaningfully involved with other people. They have things they want to do in life." History is full of such people who remain vital into advanced old age. Pablo Picasso, Arturo Toscanini, and Albert Schweitzer were all active and creative into their eighties. Goethe wrote his masterpiece, *Faust*, when he was past eighty, and Konrad Adenhauer was chancellor of Germany at eighty-seven.

Such vitality need not be accompanied by perfect physical health. In *Anatomy of an Illness*, Norman Cousins recounts a visit with pianist, conductor, and cellist Pablo Casals when the musician was almost ninety. It was clear to Cousins that Casals was probably suffering from arthritis, and he detected emphysema in Casals's labored breathing. The morning Cousins arrived, the stooped old man shuffled from his bedroom to the piano, his hands swollen and his fingers clenched.

"I was not prepared for the miracle that was about to happen," Cousins wrote. "The fingers slowly unlocked and reached toward the keys like the buds of a plant toward sunlight. His back straightened. He seemed to breathe more freely. Now his fingers settled on the keys." First came Bach and then Brahms, and as Cousins watched, the old man's body gradually grew more supple and graceful. When the music was over, there was no shuffle in the musician's step when he walked to the breakfast table, ate a good meal, and then went for a walk on the beach. This story may suggest the health-giving powers of music. More than this, it suggests how doing what you love can animate and invigorate your whole person, even into advanced old age.

Death and Healing

Psychologist Joan Borysenko tells a story about her mother's death in the Boston hospital where Borysenko was working. The eighty-one-year-old woman had been suffering from emphysema and internal bleeding and was clearly in her last hours. The family had gathered at the bedside, but suddenly the patient was no longer there. The doctors had whisked her off for a special nuclear medicine scan to discover the source of the bleeding. Back in the hospital room, the family waited and waited. Finally, the other family members said to Borysenko, "You work in this hospital. Go rescue her."

"So I went storming down to nuclear medicine," Borysenko recalled, "and I said, 'Give me my mother.'" But the doctors were reluctant. Even though the woman was clearly dying, the doctors insisted they needed to identify the source of her bleeding. "We need to establish a diagnosis."

At that, Borysenko's mother wearily raised herself on one elbow from the exam table. "You want a diagnosis? I'm dying. That's your diagnosis," she said. To Borysenko, the story is a testament to both her mother's sense of humor and the medical system's inability to know when to quit with dying patients. "To take someone away from loved ones to do final tests, to put them through the physical discomforts of the tests, and to rack up the medical bills: This verges on malpractice. Sometimes rather than trying to prolong life, it is time to allow a person to simply die."

Modern medicine has a prejudice against letting people die. The system is concerned primarily with curing, not with healing, and death is seen as the ultimate defeat, the moment beyond which no cure is possible. Preoccupied with cure, medicine often misses—or even frustrates—the healing that may go on around death: the affirmation of love and commitment within families, the focusing of values and movement toward peace as earthly existence nears an end.

DEATH, SPRITUALITY, AND HEALING

For many people the awareness of death sharpens their spiritual consciousness while increasing their appreciation of life and its mysteries. "So much in our society tries to get us to forget that life as we are conscious of it has an end," said brother Tolbert ("Toby") McCarroll, a lay Roman Catholic monk at the Starcross Community in rural northern California. "But I think that only if you understand there is going to be an end can you really plunge into the now and not take it for granted." Brother Toby and the community's three lay sisters — sister Marti Aggeler, sister Julie De Ross, and sister Cecilia Le — are more aware than most people that life is precious and can be fleeting. Since 1986 they have opened the community to six babies infected with the AIDS virus, adopting these children into their lives and family. So far, two of these children have died. The community also has established a model program for the humane health care of thirty children with AIDS in Romania.

The Starcross Community sits on six acres of rolling farmland. Brother Toby, sister Marti, and sister Julie established their religious community in 1974. All were seeking a greater sense of authenticity and spirituality in a simple, rural life. (Sister Cecilia joined them in 1992.) "Originally the idea was to move to the country and grow our own food and live the simple life of work and prayer," sister Marti said, "but it didn't quite work out that way. We kept getting involved with children." First there were foster children. Then, just as the last foster child was getting ready to graduate from high school, the community adopted a baby, named David, now seven years old. It was at about this time that the community learned that child welfare workers were unable to find homes for babies with AIDS whose mothers could not keep them. "Because we were in the process of bonding to David," said sister Marti, "we just couldn't bear the thought that there were children who had no home."

In the children, sister Marti and the others have discovered that spiritual richness they sought. According to brother Toby, "It's a lot easier for us to find what we're looking for spiritually in the children than it is sitting under a tree meditating. You look into a child's eyes, you see God. When you hold a child who is dying, you know you are in the presence of whatever mystery there is in life."

This mystery — what brother Toby calls God, or "the sacred dimension in life" — is central to his personal concept of healing. "The sacred dimension is like an offering of grace," he said. "It says to us, stop, take a breath, rest a little, consider what is really important. I think resting in the hands of God is the most fundamental kind of healing there is. That does not mean that if I have a cold and I think right, I'm going to get rid of the cold. That's not God's way. It means that I can be a whole person while I'm dying of AIDS. I can be a whole person no matter what kind of sickness I have. Our hope is to harmonize with a sort of fundamental sense of life. In that harmonization we are healed."

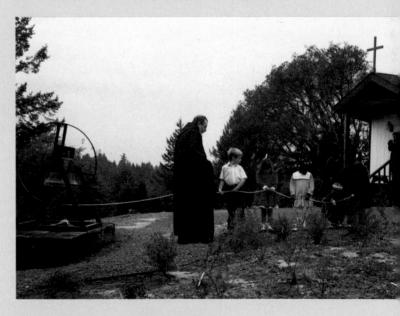

At Starcross Community in rural northern California, some of the children help brother Toby ring the bell before chapel service.

The AIDS quilt has become a vital spritual symbol through which loved ones can be mourned, and mourners can be healed and supported by others. As displayed in Washington, D.C., in October, 1992, the quilt contained twenty-thousand panels, each with a name and a tribute to a person who has died, and was ten times larger than in 1987, when it was first displayed.

Western medicine is uneasy with the idea of death, as is Western culture as a whole. It is often said that we live in a death-denying culture, but it is not so much that we deny death as that we try to ignore it. Death has been pushed to the margins of our culture. We'd rather not think about it, and we'd certainly rather not talk about it. More than sixty-seven euphemisms for death have been catalogued, including *passed on*, *expired*, *succumbed*, and *perished*. We use such expressions to distance ourselves from the reality of death.

Why are we so uneasy with death? On the one hand, we are bombarded with images of death—especially violent death—from movies and television. On the other hand, few of us see the real thing. In many cultures people die at home, surrounded by relatives who then lovingly prepare the body for burial or cremation. In our culture, death more often comes in hospitals or nursing homes. It is hard to understand that death is a part of life when the only death you will encounter may be your own.

We are also uneasy about death because of its meaning in our society. Just as cure-oriented medicine views death as the ultimate defeat, a materialistic philosophy sees it as the absolute end of the person. If we are not in any way larger than our physical bodies, then death must be a meaningless annihilation and life ultimately tragic.

The death of a loved one or the contemplation of our own death focuses our attention on spiritual issues, such as the purpose and meaning of life. For example, the AIDS epidemic has spurred a resurgence of spirituality in the male homosexual community, which has suffered disproportionately from the disease. Death touches these men dozens of times each year, and they have been encouraged to seek out some "invisible means of support." In gay communities around the country, church attendance is soaring and new churches are being formed. The AIDS quilt—in which each panel of which contains a name and a tribute to someone who has died—has become an important spiritual symbol, facilitating grief and healing wherever it is unfurled. The quilt offers a symbol around which individual losses can be mourned and individual mourners can be supported and comforted by a loving community.

In facing the questions of meaning surrounding death, many people in many cultures have come to believe that there is a spiritual presence that survives death—that moves on to another dimension or another earthly existence. Stephen Levine, a teacher of meditation and author who has worked extensively with the terminally ill, calls this belief "that sense of endlessness, or edgelessness, within." But whether you believe that death is the end of a human spirit or simply another step in its journey through time and space, the awareness of death intensifies life's meaning. If we were never going to die, why would we care about how we lived? If time were never to run out, how would we decide what was important and what was not? Death is thus a powerful spiritual force, a constant reminder that every moment is to be considered and appreciated, because it can never be lived again.

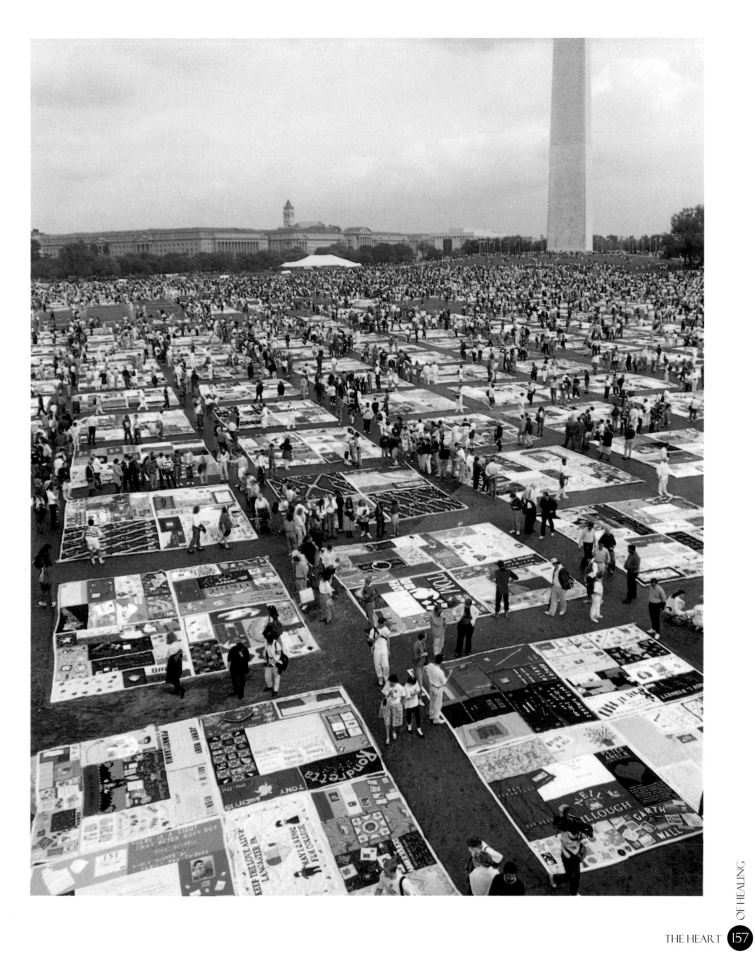

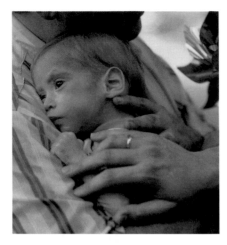

TOWARD A NEW HEALTH-CARE SYSTEM

In recent years fewer and fewer people have been satisfied with the American health-care system. One of the complaints is the expense—more than $2.5 billion each day. Total medical costs now consume more than 12 percent of the nation's gross domestic product, double the percentage spent on health in 1965. In 1992, the federal government alone spent $290 billion on health. These costs are driving medical care beyond the budgets of many Americans. In 1992, the average American household spent $8,000 on health care, about a third of that through state and local taxes. At the same time, unemployment and changing work patterns have disrupted long-standing models of health insurance coverage, leaving one in three Americans to pay for most of their health costs out of their own pockets. Too many families now live with the fear that a single catastrophic illness could lead to irreversible poverty.

It is also clear that the nation as a whole does not seem to be getting much health from its health-care dollar. Total mortality rates for all diseases have for the most part remained unchanged for thirty years, while health-care spending as a percentage of gross national product has more than doubled. Although mortality rates dropped substantially in the early decades of this century, it is widely understood that this was more the result of improved public health conditions, nutrition, and living

While the AIDS quilt gives people the opportunity to grieve for loved ones lost to AIDS, many turn to support those living with the disease. Above and below: These children with AIDS were adopted and became part of a caring, nurturing family.

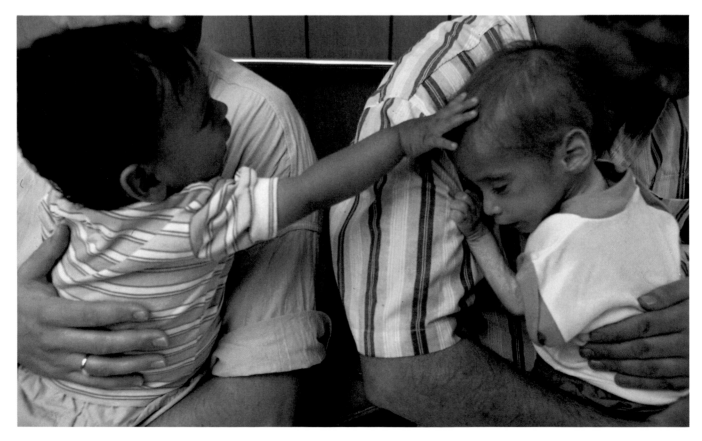

standards than of technological advances. Most of the decrease in deaths from infectious diseases, for example, occurred *before* the introduction of antibiotics in the 1950s.

Proposals for overhauling the nation's health-care delivery system abound. Some people believe the nation needs a fully paid national health-care system, such as those in Canada and Great Britain. Others espouse a plan based on "managed competition," in which private health providers and insurance companies are coordinated under close government supervision. But such plans will prove only palliative if they ignore the interplay between mind, body, and spirit that lies at the core of healing. Modern medicine does not need to be reorganized as much as it needs to be transformed—reconnected to nature, community, and family; reoriented toward a larger sense of health than the simple absence of disease. A pure system of "fix-it" medicine that seeks to cure every disease and ultimately to defeat death is more expensive than we can afford, not only in dollars but in human suffering.

There are several ways in which medicine and the approach to health could be changed to reflect the knowledge at the heart of healing. Some of the following changes are already under way.

A commitment to treat people, not diseases. Until the seventeenth century, Western medicine focused on the internal balance of bodily humors and each patient's unique complex of symptoms. As science came to associate specific diseases with these symptoms, the emphasis shifted from the individual patient to the disease itself. Lost in the process was the unique context in which the disease was experienced by the patient—what the disease meant to the patient and how it might extend from, and affect, the patient's life. A renewed medicine would return the patient decisively to the center of the system. Instead of asking, "What is wrong with this person and how can it be fixed?" physicians and other healers would ask, "Who is this person, and how can he or she be helped to achieve maximum health?" This formulation shifts the emphasis from disease to health. It no longer centers on what medicine can do for patients but on what patients, with medical help, can do for themselves.

In some ways, medicine has already begun moving toward this goal. Beginning in the 1950s, a new concern for medical ethics and patients' rights led to more patients taking control of their medical fate. In the 1960s and 1970s, patients gained the right to informed consent to medical treatments and procedures. "Living wills" evolved, through which patients could express their wishes concerning heroic life-prolonging treatments. More recently, the public's dissatisfaction with the impersonality of modern medicine has led to medical school training programs in doctor-patient relations, and some state medical boards are adding questions concerning patient sensitivity to licensure exams. In some medical schools, students check into a hospital overnight, to learn for themselves what an intravenous needle feels like and the difficulties of using a bedpan.

Accumulating evidence is showing that attention to the emotional impact of illness can directly affect healing. During one week, researchers videotaped the patient interactions of sixty-nine physicians, some of whom had received special training to help them empathize and listen to patients' emotional complaints. The researchers evaluated the emotional condition of each patient before the doctor's visit and then followed up by phone for several months. Of the 340 most distraught patients at the time of the initial visit, those who saw the specially trained doctors were found to suffer significantly less distress even six months later.

Taking account of patients' emotional needs can also save money, as shown by a study of elderly hip fracture patients at Mt. Sinai Hospital in New York and at Northwestern Memorial Hospital in Chicago. During one year, patients admitted with hip fractures received only standard psychiatric consultation (psychiatrists were called if staff noted psychiatric problems). The next year, every patient received a psychiatric evaluation on admission and counseling if needed. On average, these patients left the hospital two days earlier than the patients who had received only the "standard" psychiatric care, representing an average savings per patient of about $1,300.

A reassessment of technology. New technologies are responsible for much of the recent increase in medical costs. Diagnostic scanners, monitoring equipment, and x-ray and ultrasound technologies all provide information that helps some patients some of the time. Other patients may be helped by organ transplants, artificial organs, and new drugs. At the same time, not all medical technologies deliver as promised, and some may create more ill health than they cure or prevent. One federally commissioned study found that less than half the drugs sold between 1938 and 1962 were effective against the diseases for which they were prescribed. Another study that looked at a broad range of modern medical and surgical innovations found that only half offered improvements over standard treatments.

The public has learned some of the implications of medical technology through personal stories told in the media. Among these are the "right-to-die" cases, such as that of the twenty-one-year-old New Jersey woman named Karen Anne Quinlan, whose parents fought a ground-breaking legal battle to disconnect the young woman's life-support systems after she mysteriously went into a deep, vegetative coma. Another case is that of Dr. Barney Clark, a Seattle dentist who was implanted with an artificial heart in December 1982. Before dying of overwhelming infection 112 days later, Clark suffered seizures, lung failure, kidney disease, gout, intestinal ulcer, and nose bleeds and had to undergo surgery to replace a failing heart valve. Such cases contribute to the growing sense that while expensive medical technology may save human lives, it also can profoundly endanger human dignity. And such life-prolonging technology *is* expensive. Twenty-eight percent of the $70 billion spent by Medicare in 1985 went to people during their last year of life—and 30 percent of that $70 billion was spent during the last month of life alone. Each year an estimated $100 million is spent keeping comatose persons like Karen Anne Quinlan alive.

That so much should be spent on medical measures to keep someone alive while many other members of society go without basic medical

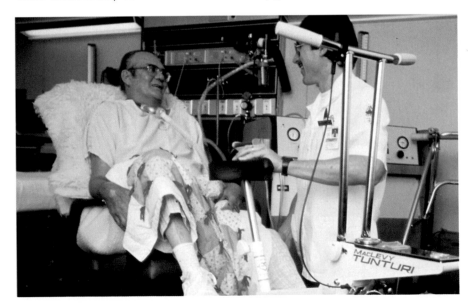

Through highly publicized cases, many Americans are beginning to understand that medical technologies can produce suffering as well as relieve it. Artificial heart patient Barney Clark suffered seizures, multiple organ failures, and bleeding problems before succumbing to overwhelming infection after 112 days.

services is the central ethical dilemma of the health-care crisis. Once life-saving technologies are developed, it is almost certain they will be used. Deciding which technologies to develop—to offer the greatest good for the greatest number at the most reasonable cost—will be a central issue as the nation struggles toward a truly sustainable health-care system.

A new openness to therapies. In January 1993, a national survey published in the *New England Journal of Medicine* reported on the use of "unconventional" health therapies by Americans. The survey cast a wide net, questioning respondents on the use of everything from massage, diet and vitamin regimes, and folk remedies to such mind-body techniques as relaxation, biofeedback training, imagery, and hypnosis, as well as such long-standing therapeutic approaches as acupuncture, chiropractic manipulation, and homeopathic medicine. The survey attracted much media attention, mostly for its key finding that, in a given year, approximately a third of all Americans will employ some treatment seen by the majority medical community as unconventional. The most commonly used therapies (other than exercise and prayer) were relaxation techniques, chiropractic manipulation, and massage.

Respondents seemed to select carefully both when and for which ailments they sought alternative treatments. Every respondent suffering from a serious disease (cancer, diabetes, hypertension) had consulted a conventional medical doctor, while perhaps pursuing alternative therapies as well. The most common complaints for which alternative therapies were sought were those that conventional medicine has been least successful in "curing": musculoskeletal pain, headache, back problems, insomnia, depression, anxiety, and arthritis. The picture that emerges from this study is of educated respondents (and, according to the survey, most of the respondents who used unconventional therapies *are* educated) making choices about their own health. Weighing the benefits and risks of the various therapies, they had decided which therapies might alleviate a specific condition or promote long-term health.

Despite this deliberateness, an editorial in the same issue of the *New England Journal of Medicine* deprecated many of the alternative treatments Americans had chosen. "Many of the relaxation techniques, massage therapies, special diets, and self-help groups could be considered to be lifestyle choices more than therapeutic interventions," the editorial opined. Other therapies were singled out as being "patently unscientific," including chiropractic, herbal medicine, homeopathy, and acupuncture—although the editorial did grant that such therapies are sometimes recommended by, or even delivered by, physicians. Two assumptions in this editorial cut to the heart of the transformation needed in our view of health and healing. First, it is clear from both traditional knowledge and the new mind-body research that "lifestyle choices" *are* therapeutic interventions. Nothing affects life that does not also affect health. This is especially true when people gain a sense of control and self-efficacy through the choices they make about health promotion, health

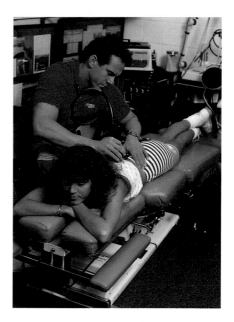

A recent survey revealed that in a given year one in three Americans will employ some "alternative" health therapy.

Among these techniques are physical treatments such as chiropractic manipulation.

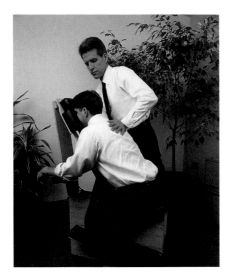

A company may use "alternative" health promotion techniques to improve the health and efficiency of workers. Shown here is a massage session at the offices of a software corporation.

maintenance, and healing. Second, the editorial's characterization of some unconventional treatments as "unscientific" misses an important point: Many of these treatments seem to work for some people some of the time, which is also true of conventional medicine. Anyone who has watched surgery performed under acupuncture anesthesia—watched surgeons open the skull of an awake, relaxed, and communicating human being—can have little doubt that the treatment works, at least for anesthetic purposes. Homeopathy, chiropractic manipulation, and some herbal therapies also seem to work for some people.

We need a system for evaluating treatments based first on efficacy. We should ask first, "Have people consistently reported, over a long period of time, that this treatment works?" If the answer is yes, we should take this testimony as one type of evidence of effectiveness—whether or not the treatment can be explained to Western scientific satisfaction. The world will continue to be full of healing mysteries, since there will always be physiological capabilities, human qualities, and spiritual forces that we cannot measure.

A new view of prevention. It is better to prevent a disease than to try to treat it, and there is ample evidence that many Americans understand this. We strive to preserve health and prevent disease with inoculations, vaccinations, a healthy diet, exercise, and safe-sex practices—and to keep abreast of each new ingredient added to the ever-evolving recipe for good health. But society has decreased its support and resources for prevention even as spending for heroic, death-defying treatments increases. Nothing represents this trend as dramatically as the disparity in the money spent to prevent premature births and to care for premature babies. Money for infant, child, and maternal health programs for the poor dropped steadily in the 1980s. This drop has led to higher rates of prematurity and related developmental disorders, such as cerebral palsy and mental retardation. The savings gained in cutting money for prenatal programs are dwarfed by the costs of caring for the premature babies. It is estimated that every dollar spent on prenatal care reduces later hospital and social expenses by almost $11, and that California alone could save $346 million a year by providing prenatal care to women who now go without it.

In general, public resources have been shifted from services that support the health of new babies to services that preserve old people in their last months of life. Technological medicine eats up so much of the health-care dollar that preventive programs are short-changed. In addition to prenatal programs for poor women, other services that were recently cut include teenage family planning, health exams for low-income children, and immunization against infectious disease.

In addition to restoring such preventive programs, we must develop a new model of prevention that takes into account the influences of emotions, attitudes, and social context on health. This may mean encouraging people to engage in daily meditation or relaxation exercises to relieve stress or promote a sense of control, or it may mean a rearrangement of priorities to create a sense of balance, purpose, and wholeness in life. There is no single road to health. Each person finds his or her own path through work, family, leisure, and community activities.

One obstacle to extending prevention into the emotional and social realm is the skeptical attitude of health insurers. Although many patients enjoy only minimal benefits from coronary bypass surgery for heart disease, many health plans cover the $30,000 expense of the operation. Very few health plans, however, will spend a few hundred dollars for a program of counseling, relaxation instruction, and lifestyle change that might prevent the progression of—or even reverse—the disease.

But true disease prevention means more than simply plugging mind-body techniques into the health-care system. We should also embrace the forces that support health—forces in nature, the family, and society. For example, we cannot ignore the impact of the environment on health. Humans evolved over hundreds of millions of years to live under a specific set of environmental conditions. During the last few hundred years modern technologies have begun to alter those conditions in dramatic ways that stress and endanger human health, resulting in air and water pollution, global warming, ozone depletion, population growth, the accumulation of carcinogens in the food chain.

Our health is also threatened by the poverty and hopelessness in our society. Poor and uneducated people run a greater risk of disease, and this has been true throughout the twentieth century. How can we inoculate children against pessimism if their families are poor, their schools rundown, and their lives circumscribed by failure? How can we encourage optimism in the homeless or a sense of purpose in the jobless or support social connectedness without supporting families?

The new health-care system should be directed not only toward preventing disease but toward preventing the social conditions that cause disease. Feeling in control is important to health. Creating a society in which the poor and disenfranchised could take control of their destinies would do more to improve the nation's overall health than updating every piece of death-defying technology in every intensive care unit in the land.

A true health system, as opposed to a simple medical system, would pay attention to the needs of people in every sense and would recognize that true health is based on self-worth, connectedness, and purpose. It would recognize that health policy is also child-care policy and welfare policy and education policy and employment policy. Beyond this, it would recognize that true health will never be achieved without a transformation of society. So much of what we need for health is missing from our lives. Only when we recover a sense of purpose as a people, a sense of community, a sense of meaning rooted in more than wealth will we learn to live without the fear of death. If each of us takes responsibility for our own health, we will gradually build a society that is not only healthy, but whole.

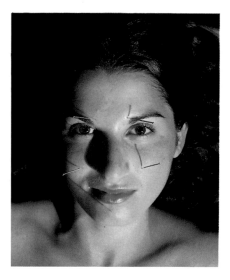

While some physicians decry alternative treatments as "unproved," a few of the techniques, such as acupuncture, have been used effectively for thousands of years.

The oldest and largest organization of its kind, the Institute of Noetic Sciences (IONS), founded in 1973, is a research foundation, an educational institution, and a membership organization with thirty thousand members worldwide.

The word *noetic* is derived from the Greek word *nous*, for mind, intelligence, and transcendental knowing. The "noetic sciences" bring the full range of diverse modes of knowing to the interdisciplinary study of consciousness, the mind, and human potential. Research topics at the Institute range from mind-body health and healing, meditation, and exceptional human abilities, to emerging paradigms in science, business, and society. The Institute does not conduct research internally, but provides seed grants for scientific and scholarly research by others, organizes lectures, sponsors conferences, and publishes books, a quarterly journal, research reports, and monographs by leading scientists, philosophers, and scholars. It also publishes a quarterly newsletter and a periodic annotated catalog of books and tapes and supports a variety of networking opportunities, member research projects, and local group activities.

The Central Role of Research

Research informs the Institute's work. As a foundation, the Institute awards seed grants, thereby establishing fruitful relationships with researchers. These relationships build and sustain connections to key organizations that are doing work in the field of consciousness studies. A stimulating cross-fertilization of ideas results from these partnerships, enlivening the entire organization not only with scientific rigor and scholarly integrity, but also with the creativity, vision, and hope that inevitably accompany the exploration of new ideas. Finally, research provides balance and legitimacy to a field that otherwise can too easily be reduced to misunderstood superficial beliefs and popular "self-help prescriptions."

The research strategy is to support carefully selected ideas and individuals who are judged to be both at the forefront of and significant to the understanding of consciousness. The strategy includes these key elements:

- identifying these ideas and individuals
- providing them with modest seed grants
- linking them to other researchers
- providing them with a safe forum for wide-ranging discussions
- offering them recognition and legitimacy by publishing their work
- providing them with opportunities to speak
- assisting them in making their work accessible to an informed public

The research focus is threefold: emerging world views, applied research derived from an unfolding understanding of consciousness, and more fundamental research regarding the nature of consciousness.

Emerging world views It seems almost trite to say that society is undergoing a profound transition. The Institute has been addressing this transformation for two decades, and today it continues to occupy a central place in research efforts. Unlike almost any other institution in our society, the Institute is addressing social change at the level of world view, beliefs, and values. It is inquiring into the process of transformation at the individual level, for organizations, and for key sectors of society (business and science). The Institute's work is based on a belief that this transformation is fundamentally about how science and spirit can be integrated, leading to world views that include such integrative concepts as "sustainable development" and "deep ecology."

Applied research areas The second focus is applied research areas that are particularly relevant to emerging world views and an understanding of consciousness. Foremost among these has been work in health and healing. IONS has funded research in imagery, biofeedback, psychoneuroimmunology (the role of the mind, emotions, beliefs, and personality in physical health), the role of spirit, the importance of "connection" (family, community, and, today, support groups), and the broad concept of health. Documenting and attempting to understand spontaneous remissions is an area of intense focus.

Altruism has been a research interest because it appears to be a natural outcome of personal transformation and because research in healing suggests that altruism positively affects health. The role of consciousness in human performance of all kinds has been another subject of inquiries. Studies have explored peak performance in athletics and the workplace, remote viewing, psychokinesis, and channeling.

The Institute has maintained a long-standing research program into different states of consciousness. Consciousness has been altered by various means in nearly every culture for purposes of healing, gaining access to knowledge not available in a normal state, gaining guidance in making life decisions in harmony with a source other than ego, and escaping from our dominant reality. Meditation is one of the Institute's current research areas. A redefinition of health and healing also involves a redefinition of death—the role of spirit in our lives, and after the death of the physical body, is a long-standing and current research interest of IONS.

The nature of consciousness The third focus of research is the field of consciousness itself. Work is focused on consciousness in traditions such as the Tibetan, as well as on recent Western scientific theories arising from quantum physics, biology, and the neurosciences. The Causality Project, a current major program, involves leading Western scientists, including two Nobel laureates, who are questioning the metaphysics of Western science based on challenges arising from the Western sciences themselves. Research into consciousness for more than twenty years points out the inadequacies of our Western scientific paradigm and strongly confirms the need to identify a suitable answer to the question of how knowledge is validated in subjective areas. The Institute believes that the time is opportune to forge alternative assumptions, indeed, a new epistemology that offers the tools to strengthen inquiries into consciousness, mind, spirit and related areas.

The Role of Research in Membership at IONS Past progress is proof that research helps legitimate promising new fields of inquiry. For Institute members, it also provides validation and grounding,

supporting them as they make vital connections between theories, exciting ideas, and the application of these ideas in daily life. This grounding provides an essential element of practicality for what would otherwise be an extremely esoteric endeavor.

The advancement of consciousness is an individual matter; we know that our membership includes individuals at the forefront of positive social change—committed to their own development and to societal transformation. In partnership with members, the Institute explores both the inner dimensions of human experience and the implications of consciousness research for personal and social change. Strategic partnerships with like-minded organizations and individuals expand educational opportunities, including the use of other communications media, such as radio, television, videotape, audiotape, and film. Member participation is encouraged through local member groups, computer networking, a membership directory, regional meetings, annual international conferences, member field research, surveys and focus groups, and a travel-study program.

All members receive these publications:

• The *Noetic Sciences Review*, a forty-eight-page quarterly journal that has become the leading periodical of its kind in the consciousness field.

• The *Noetic Sciences Bulletin*, a sixteen-page quarterly newsletter for member-related communications, networking, and education.

• *An Intelligent Guide to Books, Audiotapes and Videotapes*, an annotated, comprehensive mail-order catalog published three times per year.

The Institute of Noetic Sciences welcomes inquiries about any aspect of its activities. Please direct your inquiries to:

Institute of Noetic Sciences
Department HH
475 Gate Five Road, Suite 300
Sausalito, CA 94965
Telephone: 415-331-5650
Fax: 415-331-5673

Endnotes

Introduction

Page 8 Ambroise Paré (1517–1590) is reported to have had a favorite saying: "I treated him, God cured him."

Chapter One—Healing Mysteries

Page 13 Peggy McNeil's story is from letters from McNeil to the Institute of Noetic Sciences (March and August 1989); an interview with her oncologist, Dr. Darvey Fuller, in September 1992; and interviews with Caryle Hirshberg and Joan Saffa in June and July 1992. McNeil originally wrote a letter about her experience to Dr. Bernie Siegel in 1987 and later sent a copy of that letter to the Institute of Noetic Sciences.

14 Drs. Tilden C. Everson and Warren H. Cole reported 176 cases of spontaneous regression of cancer in their classic review, *Spontaneous Regression of Cancer: A Study and Abstract of Reports in the World Medical Literature and of Personal Communications Concerning Spontaneous Regression of Malignant Disease* (Philadelphia: W. B. Saunders, 1966).

14 The Remission Project at the Institute of Noetic Sciences houses the world's largest collection of reports of remission in both electronic form and hard copy. A selection of these reports, more than 1,300, is collected in Brendan O'Regan and Caryle Hirshberg, *Spontaneous Remission—An Annotated Bibliography* (Sausalito, Calif.: Institute of Noetic Sciences, 1993).

14 The Osler story comes from Sir William Osler, "The Medical Aspects of Carcinoma of the Breast, with a Note on the Spontaneous Disappearance of Secondary Growths," *American Medicine*, April 6, 1901, 17-19, 63-66.

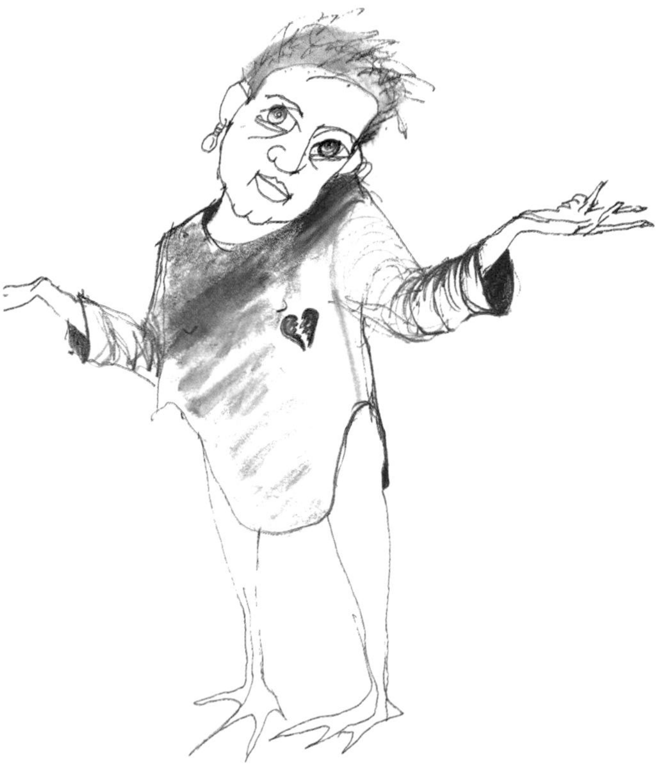

15 The story of St. Peregrine, the patron saint of cancer, and the proposal that tumors that disappear without treatment should be called Saint Peregrine tumors is reported by William Boyd, *Spontaneous Regression of Cancer* (Springfield, Ill.: Charles C. Thomas, 1966), 8.

15 The story of Bernadette Soubirous is reported by St. John Dowling, "Lourdes Cures and Their Medical Assessment," *Journal of the Royal Society of Medicine* 77 (August 1984), 634-38.

16 Vittorio Micheli's case is reported by Michel-Marie Salmon from the proceedings of the International Medical Commission at Lourdes, 1972.

18 Dowling, "Lourdes Cures," 634-38. Steve Fishman, "What a Lovely Day to Go Hunting for a Miracle," *Health* (1992), 48-59.

19 The quotations from Charles Mayo and the case history of the sixty-three-year-old woman with colon cancer is reported in an article by Mayo, "Tumor Clinic Conference," *Cancer Bulletin* 15 (1963), 78-79.

20 Information about neuroblastoma is from an article by Stephen S. Hall, "Cheating Fate," *Hippocrates* 6 (April 1992), 38. Additional information about neuroblastoma can be found in O'Regan and Hirshberg, *Spontaneous Remission*, 199-220.

20 Warren H. Cole, in the opening address at the first (and, to date, only) conference on spontaneous regression, held at the Johns Hopkins University Medical School, Baltimore, May 9–10, 1974, speculated on possible causes of spontaneous regression. Among the possible causes are hormonal influences, fever and/or infection, allergic or immune reaction, interference with the nutrition of the cancer, removal of a carcinogenic agent, unusual sensitivity to usually inadequate therapy, complete surgical removal of the cancer, or incorrect histologic diagnosis of malignancy. The proceedings of the conference are published as *Conference on Spontaneous Regression*, National Cancer Institute Monograph 44 (1976). An abstract of the conference and discussion of possible causes of spontaneous regression can be found in O'Regan and Hirshberg, *Spontaneous Remission*, 1-52, 520-30. An in-depth analysis of the role of infection in remission can be found in O'Regan and Hirshberg, *Spontaneous Remission*, 577-646.

20 Summaries of the eighteen reports of spontaneous remission associated with psychological processes can be found in Charles Weinstock, "Psychosomatic Elements in 18 Consecutive Cancer Regressions Positively Not Due to Somatic Therapy," *American Society of Psychosomatic Dentistry and Medicine Journal* 30 (1983), 151-55; Charles Weinstock, "Notes on 'Spontaneous Regression' of Cancer," *American Society of Psychosomatic Dentistry and Medicine Journal* 24 (1977), 106-10; and O'Regan

and Hirshberg, *Spontaneous Remission*, 540.

20 Only a few cases of spontaneous regression of cancer have been reported in the world's medical literature, possibly because of both the rarity of the phenomenon and underreporting. Systematic studies of spontaneous regression, therefore, are usually limited to a small number of cases. Case histories of the five cases of spontaneous regression studied by Dr. Yujiro Ikemi can be found in Ikemi, Shunji Nakagawa et al., "Psychosomatic Consideration on Cancer Patients Who Have Made a Narrow Escape from Death," *Dynamische Psychiatrie* 31 (1975), 77-92, and in O'Regan and Hirshberg, *Spontaneous Remission*, 56, 538-39.

20 A report of the findings of Van Baalen, De Vries, and Gondrie's study of six cases of spontaneous regression of cancer can be found in Daan C. Van Baalen, Marco J. De Vries, and Mayolen T. Gondrie, "Psychosocial Correlates of 'Spontaneous' Regression of Cancer," *Humane Medicine* (April 1987), 1-14.

22 The mixture that was eventually known as Coley's toxins was a combination of *Streptococcus pyogenes*, the bacteria that causes erysipelas, and *Serratia marcescens*.

22 Coley's toxins were used in 210 cases of inoperable cancers before 1940. Of 104 patients with soft-tissue sarcomas who were treated, 54 lived from five to well over twenty years. Of 60 with lymphoma, 19, or 38 percent, lived from five to twenty years, but of the 14 with breast cancer, only 2 survived five years. These statistics are quoted in Charlie O. Starnes, "Coley's Toxins in Perspective," *Nature* (May 7, 1992), 11-12. At the time Coley and others were using Coley's toxins, survival statistics were collected only by individual hospitals, if at all. To compare survival rates with Coley's toxins with survival rates with standard treatment, one should compare statistics from the same period. These statistics, however, are difficult to find. A second consideration is that the classification of sarcomas and lymphomas has changed with time. Cancers other than lymphomas are now reported by organ system, no longer by cell type. From statistics available for Stage 4 (the stage of many of the patients given Coley's toxins by Coley and others) soft-tissue sarcomas in the 1970s and 1980s (when soft-tissue sarcomas were still classified separately and thus reported separately), there was less than a 3 percent chance of surviving more than ten years. For bone sarcomas, specifically osteogenic sarcoma, the survival rate in the 1940s and 1950s was approximately 11 percent.

22 Information about Dr. William B. Coley's life and the history of Coley's toxins was collected from a number of papers and from personal communications with Helen Coley Nauts. Among these sources are Nauts, "Bacteria and Cancer — Antagonisms and Benefits," *Cancer Surveys* 8 (1989), 713-23; Nauts, "Immunotherapy of Cancer — The Pioneer Work of Coley," presented at the International Symposium on Endotoxin:

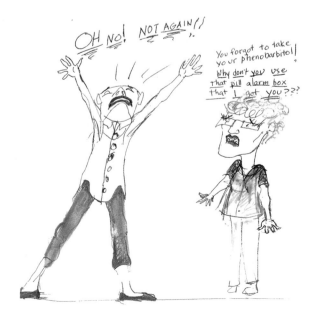

Sometimes I'm up
Sometimes I'm down

Many cancer patients find it healing to express their fears, hopes, and feelings about their illnesses through art. For years, Memorial Sloan-Kettering Cancer Center in New York has encouraged such artistic expression, and in May 1993, the hospital sponsored its fortieth patient art exhibit.

Lisa Morrongiello, who has had a brain tumor resection and received seventy treatments of radiation to the head, had a stroke in 1991, but is "feeling pretty good now." She created the art on these two pages in May 1993.

OH NO! NOT AGAIN!!

You forgot to take your phenobarbitol! Why don't you use that pill alarm box that I got you???

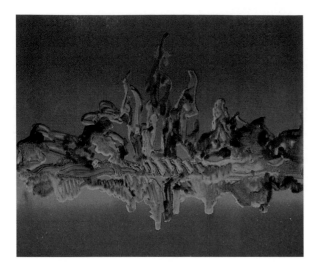

While being treated for lung cancer at Sloan-Kettering, Helen Quat was able "to happily dabble in water color and make jewelry and forget the postoperative pain." She created the monotypes *Reflections I* (above), *Patterns I* (below), and *Garden of the Deep VII* (opposite page).

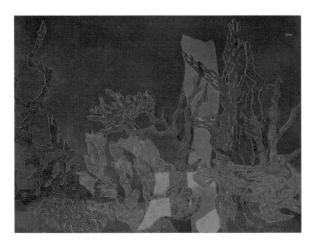

Structural Aspects and Immunobiology of Host Response, Riva del Sole, Giovinazzo, Italy, May 29–June 1, 1986; Jennifer S. Bard, "The First Stone: A Conversation with Helen Coley Nauts '25," MPS Bulletin 3 (1991); Nauts, "Coley Toxins — The First Century," presented at the International Clinical Hyperthermia Society meeting, Rome, Italy, May, 1989; and O'Regan and Hirshberg, *Spontaneous Remission*, 577-646.

23 The case of "Mr. Wright" and Krebiozen is reported in Bruno Klopfer "Psychological Variables in Human Cancer," *Journal of Projective Techniques and Personality Assessment* 21 (1957), 321-40, and in O'Regan and Hirshberg, *Spontaneous Remission*, 533.

24 Walter Cannon, neurologist and physiologist, was head of the physiology department at Harvard Medical School. He studied the effects of emotions on the autonomic nervous system, coining the terms fight or flight and *homeostasis*. According to Cannon historian Ellen Wolf, he became interested in voodoo in 1930 through Dr. Walter Alvarez. Cannon began to collect accounts from anthropologists and physicians who were in touch with aboriginal cultures and published the results of these explorations in 1942 in *American Anthropologist*. His article was reprinted in 1957 as "'Voodoo Death," *Psychosomatic Medicine* 19 (1942), 182-90. For additional work by Walter Cannon, the reader is directed to his book, *The Wisdom of the Body* (New York: Norton, 1939).

25 Kenneth M. Golden, "Voodoo in Africa and the United States," *American Journal of Psychiatry* 134 (1977), 1425-26.

25 Curt P. Richter, "On the Phenomenon of Sudden Death in Animals and Man," *Psychosomatic Medicine* 19 (1957), 191-98.

25 For additional reading: "Cultural Shock and Sudden Death" and "Stress and Sudden Death in Animals," *American Institute of Stress Newsletter* 1 (1989), 5-6.

26 The 1811 definition of *placebo* is quoted by Blair Justice, *Who Gets Sick* (Los Angeles: Jeremy P. Tarcher, 1988), 276, from an article by O.H.P. Pepper, "A Note on the Placebo," *American Journal of Pharmacy* 117 (1945), 409-12.

26 A review of fifteen studies of the placebo effect was conducted by Henry K. Beecher and reported in "The Powerful Placebo," *Journal of the American Medical Association* 159 (1955), 1602-04. This study is also cited in Michael Murphy, *The Future of the Body* (Los Angeles: Jeremy P. Tarcher, 1992), 247.

26 M. Ross and J. M. Olson, "An Expectancy-Attribution Model of the Effects of Placebos," *Psychological Review* 88 (1981), 408-37, cited in Justice, *Who Gets Sick*, 289.

27 A review of the placebo effect and surgery for angina pectoris can be found in Brendan O'Regan and Thomas J. Hurley III, "Placebo — The Hidden Asset in Healing," *Investigations* 2 (Sausalito, Calif.: Institute of Noetic Sciences, 1985), 7. Information can also be found in Justice, *Who Gets Sick*, 278-80, and in Murphy, *The Future of the Body*, 248-50.

27 Herbert T. Benson and D. P. McCallie reviewed the history of angina pectoris treatments in "Angina Pectoris and the Placebo Effect," *New England Journal of Medicine* 300 (1979), 1424-29.

27 Henry Beecher reviewed two studies in which tying off the mammary artery in surgery for angina pectoris had no greater benefit than operations in which only skin incisions were made. See Beecher, "Surgery as Placebo: A Quantitative Study of Bias," *Journal of the American Medical Association* 176 (1961), 1102-07. The two studies reviewed by Beecher were E. G. Diamond, C. F. Kittle, and J. E. Crockett, "Evaluation of Internal Mammary Artery Ligation and Sham Procedure in Angina Pectoris," *Circulation* 18 (1958), 712-13, and L. A. Cobb, G. I. Thomas, D. H. Dillard et al., "An Evaluation of Internal-Mammary-Artery Ligation by a Double-Blind Technic," *New England Journal of Medicine* 260 (1959), 1115-18.

27 Benson and McCallie, "Angina Pectoris," 1424-29, cited in Steven Locke and Douglas Colligan, *The Healer Within* (New York: E. P. Dutton, 1986), 196.

27 The study that analyzed patients' expectations about their eye operations is reported by R. C. Mason, G. Clark, R. B. Reeves, and S. B. Wagner, "Acceptance and Healing," *Journal of Religion and Health* 8 (1969), 123-42. This study is also cited in Justice, *Who Gets Sick*, 301.

27 Dr. Jerome Frank reports on the experiment performed by Dr. Hans Rehder in 1955 in *Persuasion and Healing: A Comparative Study of Psychotherapy* (Baltimore: Johns Hopkins University Press, 1973) and in Jerome Frank, "Mind-Body Relationships in Illness and Healing," *Journal of the International Academy of Preventive Medicine* 2 (1975), 46-59. The original article was written by Hans Rehder, "Wunderheilungen: Ein experiment," *Hippokrates* 26 (1955), 577-80. This study is cited in Locke and Colligan, *The Healer Within*, 198-99.

28 A randomized, controlled clinical trial to test the efficacy of two chemotherapy protocols for gastric cancer was performed at several hospitals in Britain. Four hundred and eleven patients were divided into three groups: Group A (the placebo group) received an injection of normal saline solution at three-week intervals. Group B received a five-day treatment with four chemotherapeutic agents followed by three-week injections of two chemotherapeutic agents. Group C received three-week injections of two chemotherapeutic agents. At the end of the experiment, the results and the side effects were analyzed: 34.6 percent of the placebo group reported drug-related nausea, 21.5 percent reported drug-related vomiting, and 30.8 percent reported hair loss. The results of the study are reported in J.W.L. Fielding, S. L. Fagg, B. G. Jones et al., "An Interim Report of a Prospective Randomized Controlled Study of Adjuvant Chemotherapy in Operable Gastric Cancer: British Stomach Cancer Group," *World Journal of Surgery* 3 (1983), 390-99.

28 For a summary of studies reporting physical and behavioral responses to placebos, see Sherman Ross and L. W. Buckalew, "The Placebo as an Agent in Behavioral Manipulation: A Review of Problems, Issues, and Affected Measures," *Clinical Psychology Review* 3 (1983), 457-71.

28 For a detailed summary of the 1978 study of postoperative pain in fifty-one patients who underwent dental surgery for impacted wisdom teeth, see Robert Ornstein and David Sobel, *The*

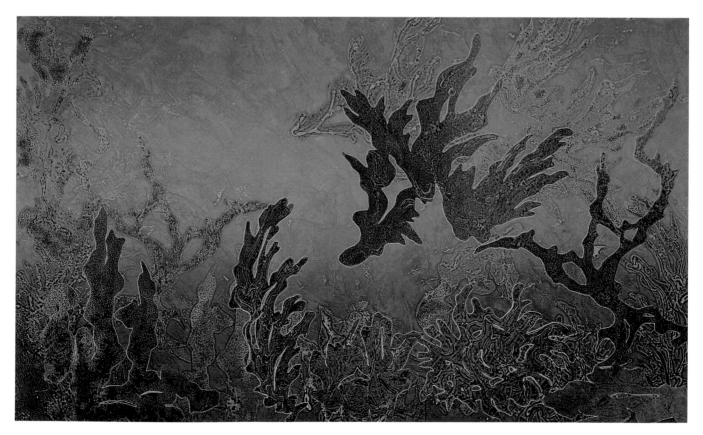

Healing Brain (New York: Simon and Schuster, 1987), 96-97. The original articles describing this study are Jon D. Levine, N. C. Gordon, and H. L. Fields, "The Mechanism of Placebo Analgesia," *Lancet* 2 (1978), 654-57; J. D. Levine, N. C. Gordon, J. C. Bornstein, and H. L. Fields, "Role of Pain in Placebo Analgesia," *Proceedings of the National Academy of Sciences* 76 (1979), 3528-31; and J. D. Levine, N. C. Gordon, R. T. Jones, and H. L. Fields, "The Narcotic Antagonist Naloxone Enhances Clinical Pain," *Nature* 272 (April 27, 1978), 826.

28 A subsequent study by Richard H. Gracely found that placebos relieved postoperative dental pain even when endorphin receptors were blocked by naloxone, suggesting that other mechanisms might have been responsible for the placebo pain relief in these patients. See Richard H. Gracely, Ronald Dubner, Patricia J. Wolskee et al., "Placebo and Naloxone Can Alter Post-Surgical Pain by Separate Mechanisms," *Nature* 306 (November 17, 1983), 264-65. In fact, placebo pain relief, like other placebo effects, is probably mediated by a multitude of mind-body connections. "There is no single placebo effect having a single mechanism and efficacy, but rather a multiplicity of effects, with differential efficacy and mechanisms" (Leonard White, Bernard Tursky, and Gary E. Schwartz, *Placebo: Theory, Research and Mechanisms* [New York: Guilford Press, 1985], 442). For a discussion of placebo analgesia and naloxone, see Priscilla Grevert and Avram Goldstein, in White, Tursky, and Schwartz, *Placebo*, 332-50

29 The history of Franz Anton Mesmer and mesmerism can be found in Norman Cousins, *Head First: The Biology of Hope and the Healing Power of the Human Spirit* (New York: Penguin Books, 1989), 169-76, and in Murphy, *The Future of the Body*, 291-95.

29 The description of a mesmeric session reported by the Royal Commission can be found in Murphy, *The Future of the Body*, 293. The original source is F. Podmore, *From Mesmer to Christian Science* (New York: University Books, 1963).

31 For more information on Dr. Spiegel's eye-roll test, see Donald S. Connery, "The Eye Roll," in *The Inner Source: Exploring Hypnosis with Dr. Herbert Spiegel* (New York: Holt, 1982), 126-41.

31 S. C. Wilson and T. X. Barber, "Vivid Fantasy and Hallucinatory Abilities in the Life Histories of Excellent Hypnotic Subjects ('Somnambules'): Preliminary Report with Female Subjects," in E. Klinger, ed., *Imagery*, Vol. 2, *Concepts, Results, and Applications* (New York: Plenum Press, 1981), 133-49. This study is described in detail in Theodore X. Barber, "Changing 'Unchangeable' Processes by (Hypnotic) Suggestions: A New Look at Hypnosis, Cognitions, Imagining, and the Mind-Body

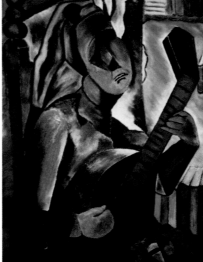

Problem," *Advances* 1 (1984), 30-34, and in Murphy, *The Future of the Body*, 317-22.

31 The results of the eye-roll test are relatively constant in an individual, suggesting that the ability to roll the eyes upward is related to biology—either it is genetically determined or is learned at a very early age. Hence, it is a biological marker for hypnotizability. This information can be found in Herbert Spiegel, "The Grade 5 Syndrome: The Highly Hypnotizable Person," *International Journal of Clinical and Experimental Hypnosis* 22 (1974), 304, and in Herbert Spiegel and Marcia Greenleaf, "Personality Style and Hypnotizability: The Fix-Flex Continuum," *Psychiatric Medicine* 10 (1992), 13-24.

31 Studies of the relationship between hypnotizability and brain function are summarized in Murphy, *The Future of the Body*, 314-16.

31 In a telephone interview with Caryle Hirshberg, Sausalito, California, May 8, 1992, Dr. Herbert Spiegel said that to express multiple personality disorder, an individual must be highly hypnotizable—it is impossible to teach someone to be highly hypnotizable since it is a biological trait related to biological markers such as eye-roll ability. Highly hypnotizable people have very mobile eyes, have a high capacity for absorption in activities, and are highly suggestible. Under the stress of abuse as a child, a highly hypnotizable child could express as a multiple or present other dissociative states, such as hysteria.

32 Cousins, *Head First*, 176-77; also Murphy, *The Future of the Body*, 297-99. James Esdaile's original work was reprinted as *Mesmerism in India and Its Practical Application in Surgery and Medicine* (New York: Arno Press, 1975).

32 The account of the amputation Dr. Esdaile performed using hypnosis can be found in Murphy, *The Future of the Body*, 299. The account was originally published by F. W. Sims in the magazine *The Englishman*, 1846, and later appeared in Esdaile's book, *Natural and Mesmeric Clairvoyance*, 1852.

32 In their review of medical literature between 1955 and 1974, Ernest and Josephine Hilgard reported on the use of hypnosis for surgical pain reduction without the use of chemical analgesics. Among the kinds of operations reported were cardiac surgery and tumor removal. See Hilgard, *Personality and Hypnosis: A Study of Imaginative Involvement* (Chicago: University of Chicago Press, 1979). The complete list of operations reported can be found in Murphy, *The Future of the Body*, 325-26.

32 Dr. Victor Rausch's account of his gallbladder surgery under hypnotic anesthesia is reported by Rausch, "Cholecystectomy with Self-Hypnosis," *American Journal of Clinical Hypnosis* 22 (1980), 124-29.

33 Dr. Frederick J. Evans's reviews of the use of hypnosis are in "Hypnosis and Pain Control," *Advances* 5 (1988), 31-39. He summarizes studies that have shown that the mechanisms whereby placebos and hypnosis mediate pain are different. In two studies comparing the effects of naloxone with acupuncture and hypnotic analgesia, researchers found that naloxone reversed the pain-relieving effects of acupuncture but not of hypnotic analgesia. See E. Goldstein and E. Hilgard, "Failure of Opiate Antagonist Naloxone to Modify Hypnotic Analgesia," *Proceedings of the National Academy of Sciences* 95 (1975), 2041-43, and D. Speigel and L. H. Albert, "Naloxone Fails to Reverse Hypnotic Alleviation of Chronic Pain," *Psychopharmacology* 81 (1983), 140-43.

33 An extensive review of the literature on hypnosis is presented by Barber, "Changing 'Unchangeable' Processes," 7-40. This is a shortened version of material that appeared in A. A. Sheikh, ed., *Imagination and Healing* (Amityville, N.Y.: Baywood Publishing, 1984). "The Case of the Sunless Sunburn" is reported by Barber, "Changing 'Unchangeable' Processes," 19, and by J. M. Bellis, "Hypnotic Pseudo-Sunburn," *American Journal of Clinical Hypnosis* 8 (1966), 310-12. The case of the hypnotized woman who was burned by an ordinary coin is reported by Barber, "Changing 'Unchangeable' Processes," 21, and by K. Platonov, *The Word as a Psychological and Therapeutic Factor* (Moscow: Foreign Language Publishing House, 1959). The case in which a hypnotized subject was burned by an ordinary pencil is reported by Barber, "Changing 'Unchangeable' Processes," 21, and by L. D. Weatherhead, *Psychology, Religion and Healing* (Nashville: Abington Press, 1952).

34 Bennett G. Braun, "Psychophysiologic Phenomena in Multiple Personality," *American Journal of Clinical Hypnosis* 26 (1983), 124-37.

34 A comprehensive review of multiple personality disorder is presented in Thomas J. Hurley III, "Multiple Personality–Mirrors of a New Model of Mind," *Investigations* 1 (Sausalito, Calif.: Institute of Noetic Sciences, 1985), 1-23.

34 Books of case accounts include Daniel Keyes, *The Minds of Billy Milligan* (New York: Random House, 1981); Hervey Cleckley and Corbett Thigpen, *The Three Faces of Eve* (New York: McGraw-Hill, 1957); and Flora Rheta Schreiber, *Sybil* (New York: Warner Books, 1974).

36 Dr. Dabney Ewin has reported several cases in which he was able to keep second-degree burns from developing into third-degree burns, which usually require skin grafting. The case of Jerry Baggett, who was burned in an explosion, is reported in *The Heart of Healing* TBS television documentary. The case of the young aluminum plant worker whose leg was burned in a vat of molten lead is reported by Barber, "Changing 'Unchangeable' Processes," 24, and by Ewin, "Hypnosis in Burn Therapy," in G. D. Burrows, D. R. Collison, and L. Dennerstein, eds., *Hypnosis 1979* (Amsterdam: Elsevier, 1979), 271-72.

36 This single-blind study was designed to determine if hypnotic suggestion could have an effect on the healing of second-degree

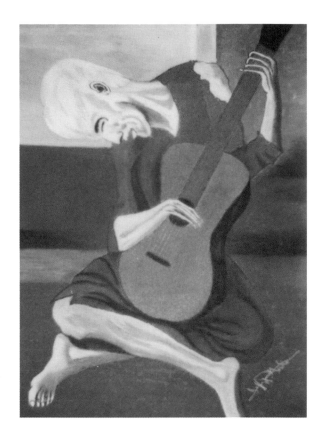

For the last seventeen years, since he was diagnosed with acute leukemia, Jeffrey Henderson has used his mind and art to "chase leukemia out of [his] body." His anger at the leukemia "was a negative force until [he] turned that anger against [his] disease." He used imagery to try to thicken his blood and to reduce high fevers from infection, and creating art was a "very strong coping mechanism." These two paintings by Henderson, *Old Man with Guitar* (above) and *Woman with Mandolin* (opposite page), were influenced by the work of Picasso.

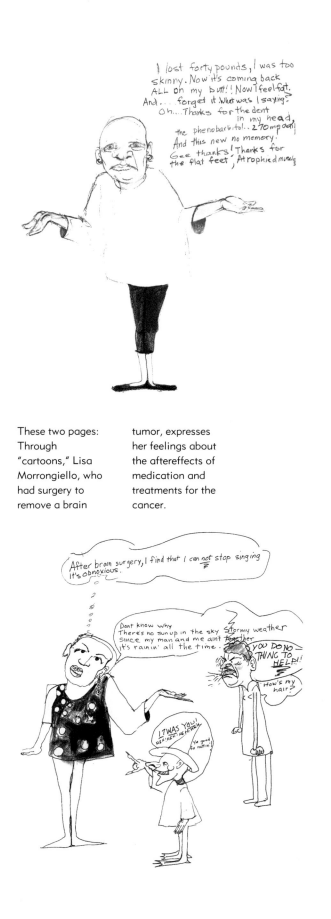

These two pages: Through "cartoons," Lisa Morrongiello, who had surgery to remove a brain tumor, expresses her feelings about the aftereffects of medication and treatments for the cancer.

burns. Each of the five subjects was hypnotized and told to increase the blood flow to the burned area on one side only. The side was picked at random by the hypnotherapist and patient. The nursing and medical staff did not know which side was chosen. Skin temperature was measured on both sides during the hypnotic induction, and two patients with burns on their hands achieved a marked difference in skin temperature on the target hand. In both these cases, the target hand healed by the sixteenth day and the other hand healed by the nineteenth day. Three of the five subjects experienced noticeable changes within three days of the hypnotherapy, and four of the five showed accelerated wound healing on the treated side. The fifth patient showed accelerated healing on both sides. This study is reported by Lawrence Moore and Jerold Kaplan, "Hypnotically Accelerated Burn Wound Healing," *American Journal of Clinical Hypnosis* 26 (1983), 16, and is cited in Murphy, *The Future of the Body*, 334.

36 A. A. Mason, "A Case of Congenital Ichthyosiform Erythroderma of Brocq Treated by Hypnosis," *British Medical Journal* 2 (1952), 422-23, cited in Murphy, *The Future of the Body*, 332. For additional cases of ichthyosis treated with hypnosis, see Barber, "Changing 'Unchangeable' Processes," 12-14.

37 Thirty studies in the last fifty years, as reviewed by David Phillips and colleagues at the University of California, San Diego, have reported the "anniversary reaction," increases in deaths around significant personal events. See D. P. Phillips, C. A. Voorhees, and T. E. Ruth, "The Birthday: Lifeline or Deadline?" *Psychosomatic Medicine* 54 (1992), 532-42.

37 Quotations attributed to Thomas Jefferson and James Monroe are reported by D. L. Mineau, "Critical Incidents in the Timing of the Moment of Death," Ph.D. dissertation, Institute of Transpersonal Psychology, 1990, 26-27.

37 The dates of the deaths of John Adams, Thomas Jefferson, and James Monroe can be found in Tim Taylor, *The Book of Presidents* (New York: Arno Press, 1972).

37 The study of occurrences of death around the Harvest Moon Festival is reported by D. P. Phillips and E. W. King, "Postponement of Death until Symbolically Meaningful Occasions," *Journal of the American Medical Association* 263 (1990), 1947-51. The researchers reviewed the death records of Chinese in California from 1960 to 1984 and correlated the data with the twenty-four-week time period centered around the Harvest Moon Festival. They found that thirty-three deaths occurred in the week before the festival, compared with the expected estimate of fifty-one, and seventy deaths occurred in the week following the Harvest Moon Festival, compared with the expected number of fifty-two. The researchers also found that mortality among old Chinese women (aged seventy-five or older) was lower the week before the festival and higher the week after the festival than in any other week in the twenty-four-week period.

37 In a study of deaths among Jewish men during the two-week period surrounding the Passover holiday, David Phillips and

Elliot King found a statistically significant decrease in the number of deaths before the holiday and an increase in the number of deaths the week after the holiday; 70 deaths occurred the week before and 113 deaths the week after Passover, compared with the expected number of 91 for both periods. This research study is published in D. P. Phillips and E. W. King, "Death Takes a Holiday: Mortality Surrounding Major Social Occasions," *Lancet* (September 24, 1988), 728-32. In both the Harvest Moon study and the Passover study, deaths from cardiovascular diseases appeared to show the most fluctuations around significant occasions.

37 Phillips and his colleagues analyzed the death certificates in California for all persons dying from natural causes between 1978 and 1990. The total number in their sample was 1,435,815, excluding persons who had undergone surgery that contributed to their death. For women of all races the researchers found that there was as much as a 3 percent greater probability of death in the week following the birthday. The results for black females showed as much as a 10.8 percent greater probability of death during this week. See Phillips, Voorhees, and Ruth, "The Birthday," 532-42, and "Fending Off Death until Birthday," *San Francisco Chronicle*, September 22, 1992, D3.

38 Yujiro Ikemi and Shunji Nakagawa, "A Psychosomatic Study of Contagious Dermatitis," *Kyushu Journal of Medical Science* 13 (1962), 335-50. Barber presents this study in detail in "Changing 'Unchangeable' Processes," 8-10.

38 O. S. Surman, S. K. Gottlieb, T. P. Hackett, and E. L. Silverberg, "Hypnosis in the Treatment of Warts," *Archives of General Psychiatry* 28 (1973), 439-41, cited in Ornstein and Sobel, *The Healing Brain*, 100. The full case is reported in O'Regan and Hirshberg, *Spontaneous Remission*, 370-71.

38 Bruno Bloch, "Ueber die Heilung der Warzen Durch Suggestion," *Klinische Wochenschrift* 6 (1927), 2271-75 and 2320-25, cited in Murphy, *The Future of the Body*, 332-33, and Barber, "Changing 'Unchangeable' Processes," 15.

38 Andrew Weil, *Health and Healing* (Boston: Houghton Mifflin, 1988), 201.

38 Lewis Thomas, *The Medusa and the Snail* (New York: Viking, 1979), 81.

39 T. Clawson and R. Swade, "The Hypnotic Control of Blood Flow and Pain: The Cure of Warts and the Potential for the Use of Hypnosis in the Treatment of Cancer," *American Journal of Clinical Hypnosis* 17 (1975), 160-69, and O. N. Lucas, "Dental Extractions in the Hemophiliac: Control of the Emotional Factors by Hypnosis," *American Journal of Clinical Hypnosis* 7 (1965), 301-07, cited in Murphy, *The Future of the Body*, 333-34.

39 Four highly hypnotizable subjects, normally reactive to tuberculin skin tests, were hypnotized daily for twelve days and given the suggestion at least five times per hypnotic induction that they would not react to the test as they had in the past. After twelve days, three of the four subjects had almost no reaction to the test and the fourth showed a small response.

This experiment is cited in Barber, "Changing 'Unchangeable' Processes," 11. The original report of this research was published by S. Black, J. H. Humphrey, and J. S. Niven, "Inhibition of Mantoux Reaction by Direct Suggestion under Hypnosis," *British Medical Journal* 1 (1963), 1649-52. In another study, a patient was hypnotized with the suggestion that one arm would not react and the other arm would react to the skin prick with tuberculin. On the arm where she was told she would receive an injection of water, there was no reaction. This research appeared in Barber, "Changing 'Unchangeable' Processes," 11. The original article was reported by A. A. Mason, "Hypnosis and Suggestion in the Treatment of Allergic Phenomena," *Acta Allergologica* 15 (1960), 332-38.

Chapter Two—Healing and Culture

Page 41 From *The Heart of Healing* television series, Turner Broadcasting Company, Inc., 1993.

42 According to the *American Heritage Dictionary* (New York: American Heritage Publishing, 1992), the word *health* comes from the Indo-European root *kailo*, from which are also derived *whole, wholesome, health, heal, holy,* and *hallow.*

43 Jean Achterberg, *Imagery and Healing: Shamanism and Modern Medicine* (Boston: New Science Library, 1985), 12.

43 Andrew Weil, *Health and Healing* (Boston: Houghton Mifflin, 1988), 47.

48 For more information on the !Kung, see Richard Katz, *Boiling*

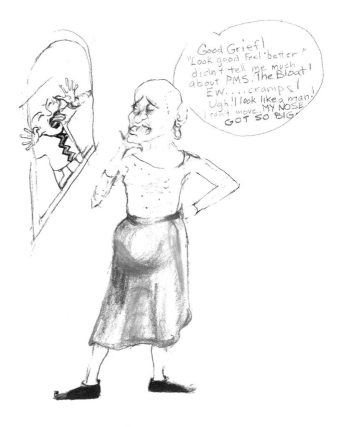

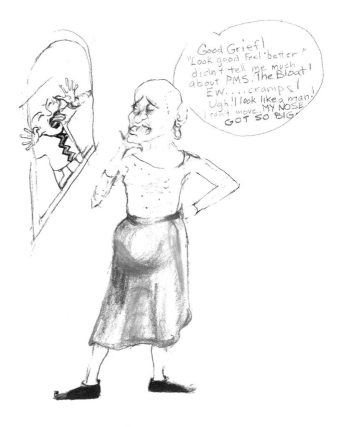Good Grief! "Look good feel better" didn't tell me much about PMS. The Bloat! EW....cramps! Ugh! I look like a man. I can't move. MY NOSE GOT SO BIG!

Energy (Boston: Harvard University Press, 1982), and Richard Katz, "Accepting 'Boiling Energy,' " *Ethos* 10 (1982), 344-67, cited in Michael Murphy, *The Future of the Body* (Los Angeles: Jeremy P. Tarcher, 1992), 271-72.

48 Information about the dream temple and Asclepios can be found in *New Larousse Encyclopedia of Mythology* (London: Prometheus Press, 1959), 163, cited in Weil, *Health and Healing*, 45.

49 For a beautifully illustrated and comprehensive history of medicine, the reader is referred to Albert S. Lyons and R. Joseph Petrucelli, *Medicine: An Illustrated History* (New York: Abradale Press, 1987), 195.

49 Quotations are from Hippocrates, *Epidemics VI*, Chapter 5, translated by W.H.S. Jones and quoted by David S. Sobel, ed., "*From The Works of Hippocrates*," in *Ways of Health* (New York: Harcourt, Brace, 1979), 194. For further information about Hippocrates, the reader is referred to Sherwin B. Nuland, *Doctors: The Biography of Medicine* (New York: Knopf, 1988), 3-30.

49 Weil, *Health and Healing*, 90.

49 Ted Kaptchuk and Michael Croucher, *The Healing Arts* (New York: Summit Books, 1987), 32.

51 In a lecture before the London College of Physicians on April 16, 1616, William Harvey presented his findings on the relationship between the heartbeat and the pulse and his theories about the circulation of blood. His treatise on the subject, *Exercitatio Anatomica de Mortu Cordis et Sanguinis in Animalibus* ("On the Movement of the Heart and Blood in Animals"), in which he concluded that the heart acted like a pump and the circulation of blood occurred in a closed system, was published thirteen years later. Harvey reached his conclusions through observations of animal anatomy and physiology. Further information about Harvey can be found in Lyons and Petrucelli, *Medicine*, 432-34, and in Nuland, *Doctors*, 120-44.

52 Descartes's discourse on the separation of mind and body is most clearly represented in his "Sixth Meditation," from *Meditations on First Philosophy Wherein Are Demonstrated the Existence of God and the Distinction of Soul from Body*, 1642. The complete quotation, as translated by Elizabeth Anscombe and Peter Thomas Geach in Descartes, *Philosophical Writings* (London: Thomas Nelson and Sons, 1971), 120, is "And thus I may consider the human body as a machine fitted together and made up of bones, sinews, muscles, veins, blood, and skin in such a way that, even if there were no mind in it, it would still carry out all the operations that, as things are, do not depend on the command of the will, nor, therefore, on the mind."

53 Sir Isaac Newton's ideas were published in *Philosophiae Naturalis Principia Mathematica*, 1687.

53 University of Texas Southwestern Medical Center, in Harper's Index, *Harper's* 285 (October 1992), 11.

53 The estimate of the cost of medical technology is from statistics of the Health Care Finance Administration, which were published in Alex Barnum, "Why Health Costs Soar So Steeply," *San Francisco Chronicle*, April 22, 1993, C1.

54 Galen wrote on the uses of medicinal plants around A.D. 160. His writings can be found in three large treatises, *On the Mixing and Efficacy of Simple Drugs* (eleven books), *On the Compounding of Drugs for Local Application* (ten books), and *On the Compounding of Drugs According to Their Kinds*. Many of his remedies were used into the twentieth century.

54 Weil, *Health and Healing*, 102-03.

54 Arnold Krochmal and Connie Krochmal, *A Guide to the Medicinal Plants of the United States* (New York: Quadrangle/New York Times Book Co., 1973).

55 Weil, *Health and Healing*, 111.

57 Louis Pasteur and Claude Bernard debated publicly and privately whether germs or the state of the bodily environment was more important in causing disease. Robert Ornstein and David Sobel, *The Healing Brain* (New York: Simon and Schuster, 1987), 29.

58 The report on the burial of Haridas was published by James Braid, the physician who coined the term *hypnosis*, in 1850 in *Observations on Trance and Human Hibernation* (London, 1850), which is based on the account of Sir Claude Wade. An account of this burial is in Murphy, *The Future of the Body*, 473-75.

58 The study of g Tummo yoga is reported by Herbert Benson, John W. Lehmann, M. S. Malhotra et al., "Body Temperature Changes during the Practice of g Tum-mo Yoga," *Nature* 295 (January 21, 1982), 234-36; John White, "An Interview with Herbert Benson, M.D.: The Principle of Maximum Mind, Insight into Extraordinary Human Potentials," *Science of Mind* (February 1988), 83; and Murphy, *The Future of the Body*, 102-03.

60 Claude Bernard, *Leçons de Physiologie Expérimentale Appliquée a la Médicine*, 2 vols. (Paris: J. B. Balliere, 1855-56), and Claude Bernard, *An Introduction to the Study of Experimental Medicine* (New York: Macmillan, 1927). A biography of Bernard was written by J.M.D. Olmstead, *Claude Bernard, Physiologist* (New York: Harper and Brothers, 1938). See also Steven Locke and Douglas Colligan, *The Healer Within* (New York: E. P. Dutton, 1986), 12.

60 "There is now good reason to hope that at least 5 percent of the estimated 1 million Americans infected with the AIDS virus may never come down with the disease," from Christine Gorman, "Are Some People Immune to AIDS?" *Time* (March 22, 1993), 49.

60 Ornstein and Sobel, *The Healing Brain*, 29.

61 Pierre Janet, along with Drs. Myers, Gibert, and others, conducted twenty-five experiments between October 1885 and May 1886 in which they tried to hypnotize subjects at a distance. They reported that they succeeded in nineteen of the twenty-five experiments. The twenty-five experiments are summarized in F.W.H. Myers, *Human Personality and Its Survival of Bodily Death*, Vols. 1 and 2 (Salem, N.H: Green, 1954). Writings by Janet include P. Janet and M. Gibert, "Sur Quelques Phenomenes de Somnambulisme," *Revue Philosophique* I and II, 1886, and P. Janet, *L'automatisme Psychologique* (Paris: Alcan, 1889). For a description of Janet's

work, see Murphy, *The Future of the Body*.

62 Franz Alexander, "Psychological Aspects of Medicine," *Psychosomatic Medicine* 1 (1939), 17-18, cited by Locke and Colligan, *The Healer Within*, 13.

63 D. Scott Rogo, *Miracles: A Parascientific Inquiry into Wondrous Phenomena* (New York: Dial Press, 1982), 274-79.

64 Hans Selye, "The General Adaptation Syndrome and the Diseases of Adaptation," *Journal of Clinical Endocrinology* 6 (1946), 117-230. See also Locke and Colligan, *The Healer Within*, 62-63.

65 René Dubos, "Introduction," in Norman Cousins, *Anatomy of an Illness* (New York: Bantam Books, 1981), 23.

66 Kaptchuk and Croucher, *The Healing Arts*, 142.

66 Weil, *Health and Healing*, 144.

66 For comprehensive and reader-friendly books about Chinese medicine, see Ted J. Kaptchuk, *The Web That Has No Weaver: Understanding Chinese Medicine* (New York: Congdon and Weed, 1983), and Harriet Beinfield and Efrem Korngold, *Between Heaven and Earth: A Guide to Chinese Medicine* (New York: Ballantine Books, 1991).

Chapter Three—Brain, Body, and Health

Page 67 O. Carl Simonton, Stephanie Matthews-Simonton, and James Creighton, *Getting Well Again* (New York: Bantam Books, 1981), 4-11.

71 For the general reader a summary of the immune system can be found in Steven Locke and Douglas Colligan, *The Healer Within* (New York: E. P. Dutton, 1986), 25-41. For current research in immunology for the general reader, see Lydia W. Schindler, *Understanding the Immune System* (Bethesda, Md.: National Institutes of Health, 1991). See also Niels Jerne, "The Immune System," *Scientific American* 229 (1973), 52-60; Peter Jaret, "Our Immune System: The Wars Within," *National Geographic* (June 1986), 702-34; and Lennart Nilsson and Jan Lindberg, *The Body Victorious* (New York: Delacorte Press, 1985).

72 S. Cohen, D. A. Tyrrell, and A. P. Smith, "Negative Life Events, Perceived Stress, Negative Affect and Susceptibility to the Common Cold," *Journal of Personality and Social Psychology* 64 (1993), 131-40; S. Cohen and G. M. Williamson, "Stress and Infectious Disease in Humans," *Psychological Bulletin* 109 (1991), 5-24; S. Cohen, D. A. Tyrrell, and A. P. Smith, "Psychological Stress and Susceptibility to the Common Cold," *New England Journal of Medicine* 325 (1991), 606-12; and David Gelman and Mary Hager, "Body and Soul," *Newsweek* (November 7, 1988), 88-97.

72 S. V. Kasl, A. S. Evans, and J. C. Niederman, "Psychosocial Risk Factors in the Development of Infectious Mononucleosis," *Psychosomatic Medicine* 41 (1979), 445-66, cited in Blair Justice, *Who Gets Sick* (Los Angeles: Jeremy P. Tarcher, 1988), 155. See also Steven F. Maier and Mark Laudenslager, "Stress and Health: Exploring the Links," *Psychology Today* (August 1985), 46.

72 A review of studies relating the activity of herpes viruses with

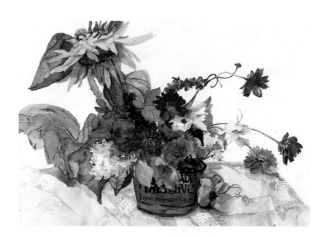

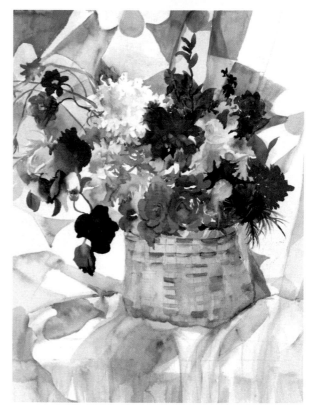

Two paintings by C. Ingrassia, a former Sloan-Kettering patient.

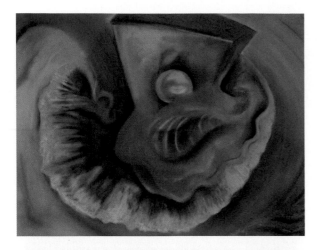

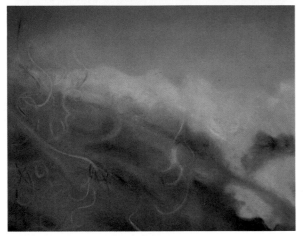

Robin Glassman, an eighteen-year survivor of adolescent Hodgkin's disease, began to paint to express, and sometimes repress, her feelings about her illness. The work on these two pages, *Oysterical Gravity* (top), *Ethereal Minuet* (bottom), and *Subaqueous Vortex* (opposite page), "is an evolution of my creative process," according to Glassman.

stress is presented by Janice K. Kiecolt-Glaser and Ronald Glaser, "The Immune System," in Daniel Goleman and Joel Gurin, eds., *Mind/Body Medicine* (Yonkers, N.Y.: Consumer Reports Books, 1993), 39-61.

72 The study with medical students was published in R. Glaser, J. K. Kiecolt-Glaser, C. Speicher et al., "Stress, Loneliness, and Changes in Herpesvirus Latency," *Journal of Behavioral Medicine* 8 (1985), 249-60; J. K. Kiecolt-Glaser, R. Glaser, E. Strain et al., "Modulation of Cellular Immunity in Medical Students," *Journal of Behavioral Medicine* 9 (1986), 5-21; and R. Glaser, J. Rice, J. Sheridan et al., "Stress-Related Immune Suppression: Health Implications," *Brain, Behavior, and Immunity* 1 (1987), 7-20.

72 The effect of divorce and separation on herpes antibodies was reported by J. K. Kiecolt-Glaser, L. Fisher, P. Ogrocki et al., "Marital Quality, Marital Disruption, and Immune Function," *Psychosomatic Medicine* 49 (1987), 13-34, and J. K. Kiecolt-Glaser, S. Kennedy, S. Malkoff et al., "Marital Discord and Immunity in Males," *Psychosomatic Medicine* 50 (1988), 213-29.

72 The study at the University of Pennsylvania and Veterans Administration Hospital was reported by L. Luborsky, V. J. Brightman, and A. H. Katcher, "Herpes Simplex Virus and Moods: A Longitudinal Study," *Journal of Psychosomatic Research* 20 (1976), 543-48, cited in Justice, *Who Gets Sick*, 156-57. See also S. E. Locke, L. Kraus, J. Leserman et al., "Life Change Stress, Psychiatric Symptoms, and Natural Killer Cell Activity," *Psychosomatic Medicine* 46 (1984), 441-53.

72 M. Kemeny, F. Cohen, and L. Zegans, "Psychological and Immunological Predictors of Genital Herpes Recurrence," *Psychosomatic Medicine* 51 (1989), 195-208.

73 J. K. Kiecolt-Glaser, J. R. Dura, C. E. Speicher, O. J. Trask, and R. Glaser, "Spousal Caregivers of Dementia Victims: Longitudinal Changes in Immunity and Health," *Psychosomatic Medicine* 53 (1991), 345-62, and *The Heart of Healing* TBS television series.

74 C. L. Fischer, C. Gill, J. C. Daniels, et al. "Effects of the Space Flight Environment on Man's Immune System: I. Serum Proteins and Immunoglobulins," *Aerospace Medicine* 43 (1972), 856, and C. L. Fischer, J. C. Daniels, W. C. Levin, et al., "Effects of the Space Flight Environment on Man's Immune System: II. Lymphocyte Counts and Reactivity," *Aerospace Medicine* 43 (1972), 1122-25, cited in Locke and Colligan, *The Healer Within*, 19.

74 A study by R. W. Bartrop and his colleagues in Australia in 1975 showed a measurable decrease in immune function after a psychologically traumatic life event, in this case, the loss of a spouse. See R. W. Bartrop, L. Lazarus, E. Luckhurst et al., "Depressed Lymphocyte Function after Bereavement," *Lancet* 1 (1977), 834-39. In 1983, Steven Schleifer and colleagues at Mount Sinai School of Medicine in New York City produced similar results in a study of men whose wives had died of breast cancer. Immune function began to recover after two months, and none of the bereaved spouses "died of grief" during the time of the studies. See S. Schleifer, S. Keller, M. Cammerino et al., "Suppression of Lymphocyte Stimulation following

Bereavement," *Journal of the American Medical Association* 250 (1983), 374-77.

74 The Russian research was published in E. A. Korneva and L M. Khai, "Effects of Destruction of Hypothalamic Areas on Immunogenesis," *Fiziol ZL SSSR* 49 (1963), 42-46, and in E. A. Korneva, "The Effects of Stimulating Different Mesencephalic Structures on Protective Immune Response Pattern," *Fiziol ZL SSSR* 53 (1967), 42-45. See also Locke and Colligan, *The Healer Within*, 46, and Robert Ornstein and David Sobel, *The Healing Brain* (New York: Simon and Schuster, 1987), 150.

75 George F. Solomon, "The Emerging Field of Psychoneuroimmunology," *Advances* 2 (1985), 11, and Locke and Colligan, *The Healer Within*, 46.

75 George F. Solomon and Rudolf H. Moos, "The Relationship of Personality to the Presence of Rheumatoid Factor in Asymptomatic Relatives of Patients with Rheumatoid Arthritis," *Advances* 1 (1984), 41-48. This article was originally published in 1965 in *Psychosomatic Medicine* and by George F. Solomon as "Emotional and Personality Factors in the Onset and Course of Autoimmune Disease, Particularly Rheumatoid Arthritis," in Robert Ader, ed., *Psychoneuroimmunology* (New York: Academic Press, 1981), 159-82.

76 Robert Ader and Nicholas Cohen, "Behaviorally Conditioned Immunosuppression," *Psychosomatic Medicine* 37 (1975), 333-

40, cited in Harris Dienstfrey, *Where the Mind Meets the Body* (New York: HarperCollins, 1991), 71ff. A review of the work in conditioned immunosuppression can be found in Robert Ader and Nicholas Cohen, "Conditioned Immunopharmacologic Effects," in Ader, *Psychoneuroimmunology*, 281-319.

77 H. O. Besedovsky, E. Sorkin, D. Felix, and H. Haas, "Hypothalamic Changes during the Immune Response," *European Journal of Immunology* 7 (1977), 325-28. Summaries of Besedovsky's work can be found in Locke and Colligan, *The Healer Within*, 55, and in Ornstein and Sobel, *The Healing Brain*, 150.

78 K. Bulloch and R. Y. Moore, "Innervation of the Thymus Gland of Brainstem and Spinal Cord in Mouse and Rat," *American Journal of Anatomy* 162 (1981), 157-66.

78 J. M. Williams, R. G. Petersen, P. A Shea, J. F. Schmedtje, D. C. Bauer, D. L. Felten, S. Y. Felten et al., "Noradrenergic and Peptidergic Innervation of Lymphoid Tissue," *Journal of Immunology* 135 (1985), 755s-65s, and D. Felten, "Sympathetic Innervation of Murine Thymus and Spleen: Evidence for a Functional Link between the Nervous and Immune Systems," *Brain Research Bulletin* 6 (1981), 83-94, cited in Locke and Colligan, *The Healer Within*, 50-51.

79 Karen Olness and Robert Ader, "Conditioning as an Adjunct in the Pharmacotherapy of Lupus Erythematosus," *Developmental*

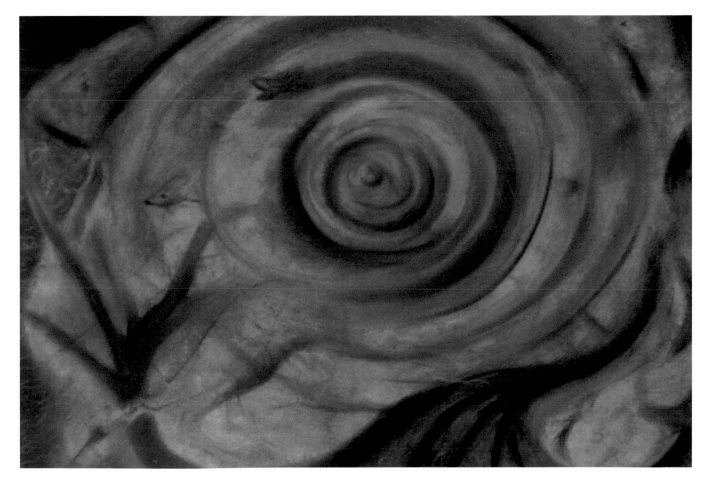

and Behavioral Pediatrics 13 (1992), 124-25.

80 Walter B. Cannon, "The Emergency Function of the Adrenal Medulla in Pain and the Major Emotions," *American Journal of Physiology* 33 (1926), 356-72, and Hans Selye, *The Physiology and Pathology of Exposure to Stress* (Montreal: Acta, 1975), cited in Locke and Colligan, *The Healer Within*, 63.

80 B. Crary, M. Borysenko, D. C. Sutherland et al., "Decrease in Mitogen Responsiveness of Mononuclear Cells from Peripheral Blood after Epinephrine Administration in Humans," *Journal of Immunology* 130 (1983), 694-97, and B. Crary, S. L. Hauser, M. Borysenko et al., "Epinephrine-Induced Changes in the Distribution of Lymphocyte Subsets in Peripheral Blood of Humans," *Journal of Immunology* 131 (1983), 1178-81.

80 The norepinephrine study is cited by Locke and Colligan, *The Healer Within*, 65-66.

80 C. B. Pert and S. H Snyder, "Opiate Receptor: Demonstration in Nervous Tissue," *Science* 179 (1973), 1011-14; C. B. Pert, G. Pasternak, and S. H. Snyder, "Opiate Agonists and Antagonists Discriminated by Receptor Binding in Brain," *Science* 182 (1973), 1359-61; and Candace B. Pert, M. J. Kuhar, and Solomon Snyder, "Opiate Receptor: Autoradiographic Localization in Rat Brain," *Proceedings of the National Academy of Sciences* 73 (1976), 3729-33. See also Rob Wechsler, "A New Prescription: Mind over Malady," *Discover* (February 1987), 53.

82 For information on brain physiology and evolution, see Floyd E. Bloom, Arlyne Laxerson, and Laura Hofstadter, *Brain, Mind and Behavior* (New York: Freeman, 1985); R. Ornstein, R. Thompson, and D. Macaulay, *The Amazing Brain* (Boston: Houghton Mifflin, 1984) and Paul MacLean, *A Truine Concept of the Brain and Behavior* (Toronto: University of Toronto Press, 1973).

82 See also Ornstein and Sobel, *The Healing Brain*, 36-42.

82 Paul D. MacLean, "Brain Evolution Relating to Family, Play, and the Separation Call," *Archives of General Psychiatry* 42 (April 1985), 405-17.

83 Lydia Temoshok and Henry Dreher, *The Type C Connection* (New York: Random House, 1992), 192, and Candace B. Pert, "Neuropeptides: The Emotions and Bodymind," *Noetic Sciences Review* 2 (1987), 13-18.

83 Working with animals, Pert, Ruff, and associates identified receptors for neuropeptides on cells in the immune system. See Candace Pert, "The Wisdom of the Receptors: Neuropeptides, the Emotions, and Bodymind," *Advances* 3 (1986), 8-16, and Candace Pert, Michael Ruff, Richard Weber, and Miles Herkenham, "Neuropeptides and Their Receptors: A Psychosomatic Network," *Journal of Immunology* 135 (1985), 820s-26s.

84 William H. Frey, telephone interview with Caryle Hirshberg, March 1993; William H. Frey II, "Not-So-Idle Tears," *Psychology Today* (January 1980), 91-92; Karen Freifold, "A Good Cry; Tears, Scientists Find, Hold Clues to Everything from Eye Disorders to General Health," *Forbes* 134 (November 5, 1984), 232-34; William H. Frey II, *Crying: The Mystery of Tears* (New York: Harper and Row, 1985); Ornstein and Sobel, *The Healing*

Brain, 43-44; and Nancy Stesin, "The Best Stress Relief (Crying)," *Ladies Home Journal* 109 (1992), 86-87.

85 J. E. Blalock, "The Immune System as a Sensory Organ," *Journal of Immunology* 132 (1984), 1067-70; J. E. Blalock, "A Molecular Basis for Bidirectional Communication between the Immune and Neuroendocrine Systems," *Physiological Reviews* 69 (1989), 1-32; E. M. Smith and J. E. Blalock, "Human Lymphocyte Production of Corticotropin and Endorphin-like Substances: Association with Leukocyte Interferon," *Proceedings of the National Academy of Sciences* 78 (1981), 7530-34; and J. E. Blalock, M. P. Langford et al., "Nonsensitized Lymphocytes Produce Leukocyte Interferon When Cultured with Foreign Cells," *Cell Immunology* 43 (1979), 197-201.

85 Norman Cousins, *Human Options: An Autobiographical Notebook* (New York: Norton, 1981).

Chapter Four—Who Gets Sick

Page 87 Material about the Army War College in Carlisle, Pennsylvania, is from *The Heart of Healing* TBS television series interviews and from James J. Gill, Virginia A. Price, Meyer Friedman, Carl E. Thoresen et al., "Reduction in Type A Behavior in Healthy Middle-Aged American Military Officers," *American Heart Journal* 110 (1985), 503-14.

87 Meyer Friedman, *Treating Type A Behavior and Your Heart* (New York: Ballantine Books, 1984), 3-6, and Gill, Price, Friedman, Thoresen et al., "Reduction in Type A Behavior," 511. For additional information, see Virginia A. Price, *Type A Behavior Pattern: A Model for Research and Practice* (New York: Academic Press, 1982).

93 William Osler, from an article in *Lancet* in 1910, in Joan Arehart-Treichel, *Biotypes: The Critical Link between Your Personality and Your Health* (New York: Times Books, 1980), 33.

93 For a review of personality and health, see Arehart-Treichel, *Biotypes*.

93 For a discussion of the relationship between hostility and Type A, see Redford Williams, "About Hostility and Type A: From Confusion to Clarification," in *The Trusting Heart* (New York: Times Books, 1989), 44-71.

95 Bernard Gavzer, "What We Continue to Learn from People Who Survive AIDS," *San Francisco Chronicle and Examiner*, January 31, 1993, 4-7.

95 The pilot study of the psychosocial characteristics of long survivors of AIDS was reported by George F. Solomon, Lydia Temoshok, Ann O'Leary, and Jane Zich, "An Intensive Psychoimmunologic Study of Long-Surviving Persons with AIDS," *Annals of the New York Academy of Sciences* 496 (1987), 647-55. See also Henry Dreher, "Are You Immune-Competent?" *Natural Health* (January/February 1992), 52-59.

96 A summary of the Precursor Study was published by Caroline B. Thomas, "Cancer and the Youthful Mind: A Forty-Year Perspective," *Advances* 5 (1988), 42-58.

98 Robert W. Levenson, Paul Ekman, and Wallace V. Friesen, "Voluntary Facial Action Generates Emotion-Specific

Autonomic Nervous System Activity," *Psychophysiology* 27 (1990), 363-84. See also Bruce Bower, "The Face of Emotion," *Science News* 128 (July 6, 1985), 12-13; Sally Squires, "The Mind Fights Back," *Washington Post*, January 9, 1985, 16; and Paul Ekman, "Expression and the Nature of Emotion," in Klaus Scherer and Paul Ekman, eds., *Approaches to Emotion* (Hillsdale, N.J.: Lawrence Erlbaum, 1984), 324-29.

99 Alice Epstein's story is from *The Heart of Healing* TBS television series and from Alice Epstein's published account of her experiences (Alice Hopper Epstein, *Mind, Fantasy and Healing*, [New York: Delacorte Press, 1989].). For more information about the Type C personality, see Lydia Temoshok and Henry Dreher, *The Type C Connection: The Behavioral Links to Cancer and Your Health* (New York: Random House, 1992).

100 Norman Cousins, *Anatomy of an Illness as Perceived by the Patient* (New York: Norton, 1979), 39.

100 The effect of laughter on blood pressure, heart rate, oxygen saturation levels, and respiratory activity is reported in W. F. Fry, Jr., and W. M. Savin, "Mirthful Laughter and Blood Pressure," *Humor* 1 (1988), 49-62, and in W. F. Fry, Jr., and P. E. Stoft, "Mirth and Oxygen Saturation Levels of Peripheral Blood," *Psychotherapy and Psychosomatics* 19 (1971), 76-84. The effects of laughter on body chemistry are reported by Lee S. Berk, Stanley A. Tan, William F. Fry et al., "Neuroendocrine and Stress Hormone Changes during Mirthful Laughter," *American Journal of Medical Sciences* 298 (December 1989), 390-96.

100 The effects of laughter on the production of antibodies in the upper respiratory track are reported by K. M. Dillon, B. Minchoff, and K. H. Baker, "Positive Emotional States and Enhancement of the Immune System," *International Journal of Psychiatry in Medicine* 15 (1985-1986), 13-18.

100 The use of laughter by health-care professionals and hospitals is reported by Jane E. Brody, "Personal Health: Increasingly, Laughter as Potential Therapy for Patients Is Being Taken Seriously," New York Times, April 7, 1988, B8. See also Norman Cousins, *Head First: The Biology of Hope and the Healing Power of the Human Spirit* (New York: Penguin Books, 1989), 140-41.

104 The Minnesota study has published a number of articles about research with identical twins reared apart. Among these articles are Thomas J. Bouchard, Jr., David T. Lykken, Matthew McGue, Nancy L. Segal, and Auke Tellegen, "Sources of Human Psychological Differences: The Minnesota Study of Twins Reared Apart," *Science* 250 (October 12, 1990), 223-28; Niels G. Waller, Brian A. Kojetin, Thomas J. Bouchard, Jr., et al., "Genetic and Environmental Influences on Religious Interests, Attitudes and Values: A Study of Twins Reared Apart and Together," *Psychological Science* 1 (1990), 138-42; and Auke Tellegen, David T. Lykken, Thomas J. Bouchard, Jr., et al., "Personality Similarity in Twins Reared Apart and Together," *Journal of Personality and Social Psychology* 54 (1988), 1031-39.

104 The story of Jerry Levey and Mark Newman and the twins named Jim was reported by Clare Mead Rosen, "The Eerie World

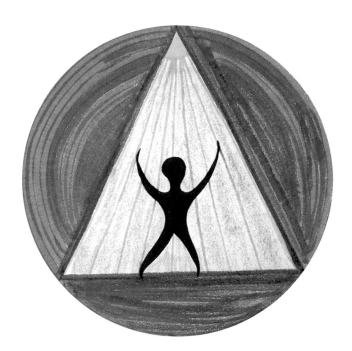

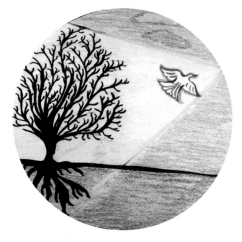

Laurie Downs, who has been in remission from cancer for five years, began to paint while she was participating in an art therapy group. These two paintings are enclosed by mandalas, a technique used in the art therapy process.

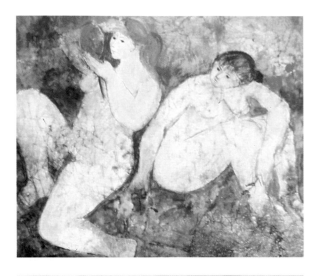

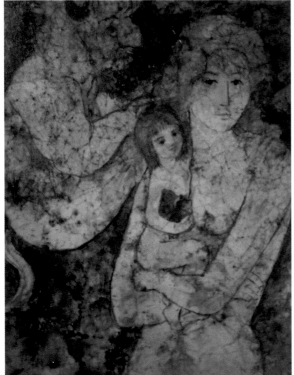

After developing cancer of the thyroid thirty-three years ago, Trudy Lanitis, previously a commercial artist, became even more involved with art, concentrating on both sculpting and painting. *Two Nudes* (top, owned by The Art Garden) and *Mother, Child, and Satyr* (bottom, owned by John Barnes) were "spiritually conceived," according to Lanitis, while she was in a meditative state, which is part of her spiritual healing process.

of Reunited Twins," *Discover* (September 1987), 36-46.

105 The subjects of this study, 259 men in job levels from middle managers to officers in a utility company, were asked to fill out questionnaires covering a period of five years to determine whether hardiness, committment, control, and challenge decreased the effects of stressful events in producing illness. See Suzanne C. Kobasa, "Stressful Life Events, Personality, and Health: An Inquiry into Hardiness," *Journal of Personality and Social Psychology* 37 (1979), 1-11, and Suzanne C. Kobasa, Salvatore R. Maddi, and Stephen Kahn, "Hardiness and Health: A Prospective Study," *Journal of Personality and Social Psychology* 42 (1982), 169-70. The study of the Illinois Bell executives was published as Maddi and Kobasa, *The Hardy Executive: Health under Stress* (Homewood, Ill.: Dow Jones-Irwin, 1984). This work is summarized in Steven Locke and Douglas Cooligan, *The Healer Within* (New York: E. P. Dutton, 1986), 82, 84, and 92.

106 Quotes are from transcripts of interviews with Janice K. Kiecolt-Glaser and Ronald Glaser from *The Heart of Healing* TBS television series.

106 The effects of marital disruption on immune function is reported by Janice K. Kiecolt-Glaser, Laura D. Fisher, Paula Ogrocki, Julie C. Stout, Carl E. Speicher, and Ronald Glaser, "Marital Quality, Marital Disruption, and Immune Function," *Psychosomatic Medicine* 49 (1987), 13-34.

106 The newlyweds study is reported by Janice K. Kiecolt-Glaser, Ronald Glaser, and William B. Malarkey, "Negative Behavior during Marital Conflict Is Associated with Immunological Down-Regulation," *Psychosomatic Medicine* (in press).

107 Madelon Visintainer's work is published in M. Visintainer, J. Volpicelli, and M.E.P. Seligman, "Tumor Rejection in Rats after Inescapable or Escapable Shock," *Science* 216 (1982), 437-39, and is described in Martin E. P. Seligman, *Learned Optimism* (New York: Simon and Schuster, 1990), 168-71. Other animal research linking stress and changes in immune measures includes V. Riley, M. A. Fitzmaurice, and D. H. Spackman, "Psychoneuroimmunologic Factors in Neoplasia: Studies in Animals," in Rober Ader, ed., *Psychoneuroimmunology* (New York: Academic Press, 1981), 31-102, and M. L. Laudenslager, S. M. Ryan, R. C. Drugan, R. L. Hyson, and S. F. Maier, "Coping and Immunosuppression: Inescapable But Not Escapable Shock Suppresses Lymphocyte Proliferation," *Science* 221 (1983), 568-70. For a popular article on stress and health, see Steven F. Maier and Mark Laudenslager, "Stress and Health: Exploring the Links," *Psychology Today* (August 1985), 44-49.

107 Ellen J. Langer and Judith Rodin, "The Effects of Choice and Enhanced Personal Responsibility for the Aged: A Field Experiment in an Institutional Setting," *Journal of Personality and Social Psychology* 34 (1976), 191-98, cited in Seligman, *Learned Optimism*, 169.

107 R. B. Shekelle, W. J. Raynor, A. M. Ostfeld et al., "Psychological Depression and 17-Year Risk of Death from Cancer," *Psychosomatic Medicine* 43 (1981), 117-25.

108 Robert Ornstein and David Sobel, *The Healing Brain* (Simon and Schuster, 1987), 132-34.

108 For additional information about human attachment, see J. Bowlby, *Attachment and Loss*, vols. 1-3 (New York: Basic Books, 1969), and M.D.S. Ainsworth and S. M. Bell, "Attachment, Exploration, and Separation: Illustrated by the Behavior of One-Year-Olds in a Strange Situation," *Child Development* 41 (1970).

109 C. Peterson, M. Seligman, and G. Vaillant, "Pessimistic Explanatory Style as a Risk Factor for Physical Illness: A Thirty-Five Year Longitudinal Study," *Journal of Personality and Social Psychology* 55 (1988), 23-28. This study is cited in Seligman, *Learned Optimism*, 179-81.

109 The studies of the baseball players are summarized in Seligman, *Learned Optimism*, 157-60.

110 L. F. Berkman and S. L. Syme, "Social Networks, Host Resistance, and Mortality: A Nine-Year Follow-up Study of Alameda County Residents," *American Journal of Epidemiology* 109 (1979), 186-204. See also J. S. House, K. R. Landis, and D. Umberson, "Social Relationships and Health," *Science* 241 (July 1988), 540-45, and J. S. House, C. Robbins, and H. L. Metzner, "The Association of Social Relationships and Activities with Mortality," *American Journal of Epidemiology* 116 (1982), 123-40.

110 Research on Japanese, Japanese-Americans, and heart disease is in M. G. Marmot and S. L. Syme, "Acculturation and Coronary Heart Disease in Japanese-Americans," *American Journal of Epidemiology* 104 (1976), 225-47, and in M. G. Marmot, S. L. Syme, A. Kagan et al., "Epidemiological Studies of Coronary Heart Disease and Stroke in Japanese Men Living in Japan, Hawaii, and California: Prevalence of Coronary and Hypertensive Heart Disease and Associated Risk Factors," *American Journal of Epidemiology* 102 (1975), 514-25. These studies are also discussed in Ornstein and Sobel, *The Healing Brain*, 125-26.

110 The concept of *amae* is discussed in Blair Justice, *Who Gets Sick* (Los Angeles: Jeremy P. Tarcher, 1988), 133. For more on amae, see L. T. Doi, "Amae: A Key Concept for Understanding Japanese Personality Structure," in T. S. Lebra and W. P. Lebra, eds., *Japanese Culture and Behavior* (Honolulu: Unversity Press of Hawaii, 1974), 145-54.

111 The Duke University study of 1,368 heart disease patients was reported by R. B. Williams, J. C. Barefoot, R. M. Califf et al., "Prognostic Importance of Social and Economic Resources among Medically Treated Patients with Angiographically Documented Coronary Artery Disease," *Journal of the American Medical Association* 267 (January 22/29, 1992), 520-24. A popular article about friendship and health is Jane E. Brody, "Personal Health: Maintaining Friendships for the Sake of Health," *New York Times*, February 5, 1992, B8-9.

111 A good review of the evidence that links social support and health can be found in S. Cohen and S. L. Syme, eds., *Social Support and Health* (New York: Academic Press, 1985). Several other articles have been published that show links between health and social support, including L. F. Berkman, "Assessing the Physical Health Effects of Social Networks and Social Support," *Annual Review of Public Health* 5 (1984), 413-32.

111 J. K. Kiecolt-Glaser, W. Garner, C. E. Speicher, G. Penn, and R. Glaser, "Psychosocial Modifiers of Immunocompetence in Medical Students," *Psychosomatic Medicine* 46 (1984), 7-14.

111 The study of 256 healthy elderly adults was reported by P. D. Thomas, J. M. Goodwin, and J. S. Goodwin, "Effect of Social Support on Stress-Related Changes in Cholesterol Level, Uric Acid Level, and Immune Function in an Elderly Sample," *American Journal of Psychiatry* 142 (1985), 735-37.

Chapter Five—Getting Well

Page 113 The Office of Alternative Medicine (OAM) was created in response to a request by Congress that accompanied the 1992 fiscal year Labor, HHS, and Education and Related Agencies Appropriation Bill, passed in October 1991, that the National Institutes of Health establish an office to evaluate alternative medical practices. Some of the practices to be investigated include diet, nutrition, and lifestyle changes; mind-body control, such as relaxation, biofeedback, imagery, and music therapy; traditional medical modalities, such as acupuncture, herbal medicine, homeopathic medicine, and Native American medicine; physical manipulation therapies, such as massage, rolfing, therapeutic touch, and Qi Gong; biological treatments, such as antioxidant, cell, and metabolic therapies; and the therapeutic use of electromagnetic fields.

114 Material about the meditation program at Dorchester High School in Boston is from videotapes and an interview with Olivia Hoblitzelle from *The Heart of Healing* TBS television series.

114 Herbert Benson began his study of transcendental meditation in about 1968. He and co-researcher R. Keith Wallace measured the physiological effects of TM, specifically to see if it could lower blood pressure. Though TM did not affect blood pressure in these experiments, they found that meditation did lower heart rates, breathing rates, and oxygen consumption and produced higher alpha brain waves. In later experiments with hypertensive people, Benson was able to demonstrate a reduction in blood pressure. In 1972, he named the response he had studied "the Relaxation Response." In 1975 he wrote *The Relaxation Response* (New York: Morrow, 1975). Wallace and Benson published a number of reports on their collaborative research, among them: R. K. Wallace, H. Benson, and A. F. Wilson, "A Wakeful Hypometabolic State," *American Journal of Physiology* 221 (1971), 795-99; R. K. Wallace and H. Benson, "The Physiology of Meditation," *Scientific American* 226 (1972), 84-90; and H. Benson and R. K. Wallace, "Decreased Blood Pressure in Hypertensive Subjects Who Practiced Meditation," *Circulation* 46 (1972), 130. For a review of the history of Benson and Wallace's work, see Harris Dientsfrey, *Where the Mind Meets the Body* (New York: HarperCollins, 1991), 25-43.

115 Quotes are from interview with Dr. Joan Borysenko from *The Heart of Healing* TBS television series.

117 Dr. Ainslie Meares, an Australian psychiatrist, has reported several cases of patients who have achieved remissions from cancer through the use of intensive meditation, among them cases of breast cancer, osteogenic sarcoma, colorectal cancer, and lung cancer. The full text of some of these case reports can be found in Brendan O'Regan and Caryle Hirshberg, *Spontaneous Remission—An Annotated Bibliography* (Sausalito, Calif.: Institute of Noetic Sciences, 1993), 549-56.

117 Doris Phillips's story is from interviews with Dr. James Suen, Dr. Stephanie Simonton, Doris Phillips, and her daughter Aven, in *The Heart of Healing* TBS television series.

117 O. Carl Simonton, Stephanie Matthews-Simonton, and James Creighton, *Getting Well Again* (New York: Bantam Books, 1981).

117 Information about imagery is from Jeanne Achterberg, *Imagery in Healing: Shamanism and Modern Medicine* (Boston: New Science Library, 1985), 14, 56, 104-07; Jeanne Achterberg and G. Frank Lawlis, *Imagery and Disease* (Champaign, Ill.: Institute for Personality and Ability Testing, 1984), 141-53; and Dientsfrey, *Where the Mind Meets the Body*, 125-42.

117 Research on imagery and its effect on the immune system is reported in Achterberg and Lawlis, *Imagery and Disease*, 141-53; G. R. Smith, Jr., J. M. McKenzie, D. J. Marmer et al., "Psychologic Modulation of the Human Immune Response to Varicella," *Archives of Internal Medicine* 145 (1985), 2110-12; and Stephanie Simonton-Atchley, G. Richard Smith, James Y. Suen, Russell W. Steele, and Ronald K. Charlton, "Psychological Modulation of Cellular Immunity in Cancer Patients: Report of Research in Progress" (research report to the Institute of Noetic Sciences).

120 Dragomir Cioroslan's story is from a videotaped interview for *The Heart of Healing* TBS television series. Cioroslan is the national resident coach of the United States Weightlifting Federation. His story was also featured in Paul Shepherd, "The Torch of Technology: The Science behind the '92 Olympics," *Omni* 14 (July 1992), 42-44, 46, and 74.

121 Information about Marilyn King is from an interview with her in Barbara McNeill, "Beyond Sports: Imaging in Daily Life; an Interview with Marilyn King," *Noetic Sciences Collection* (1985), 32-34.

122 Information about Chris Kelly is from interviews with Chris Kelly and Dr. Bernard Brucker from *The Heart of Healing* TBS television series and from J. Morrow and R. Wolff, "Wired for a Miracle," *Health* (May 1991), 64-69, 84. Additional information about Brucker's use of biofeedback for patients with spinal cord injuries and paralysis can be found in Dientsfrey, *Where the Mind Meets the Body*, 62-66, and in Bernard Brucker and Laurence P. Ince, "Biofeedback as an Experimental Treatment for Postural Hypotension in a Patient with Spinal Cord Lesion," in Johann Stoyva et al., *Biofeedback and Self-*

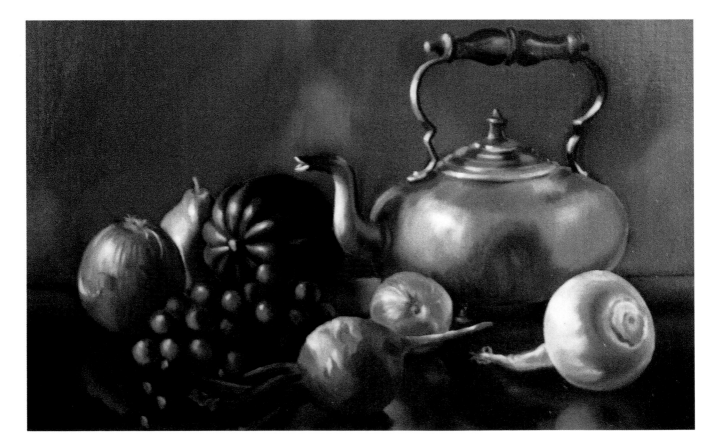

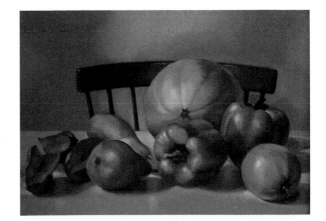

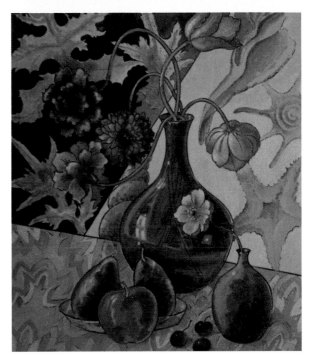

Control, 1977/78 (Chicago: Aldine, 1978).

122 Dr. Neal Miller's work with animals and the history of early biofeedback work with humans can be found in Dientsfrey, *Where the Mind Meets the Body*, 45-69, and in Harris Dientsfrey, "Neal Miller, the Dumb Autonomic Nervous System, and Biofeedback," *Advances* 7 (1991), 33-44.

124 The NASA experiments with biofeedback training for motion sickness are conducted by Dr. Patricia S. Cowings, a researcher at Ames Research Center in Mountain View, California. Information about the training is from interviews with Dr. Cowings; Mae Jemison, the astronaut who "flew" the experiment on the space shuttle, from *The Heart of Healing* TBS television series; and Patricia S. Cowings, "Autogenic-Feedback Training as a Preventive Method for Space Motion Sickness," typescript. See also "Shuttle Crew Tries Out Biofeedback: Relaxation Technique Could Help Prevent Motion Sickness in Space," *San Francisco Chronicle*, September 14, 1992, A7.

124 Eugene G. Peniston and Paul J. Kulkosky, "Alcoholic Personality and Alpha-Theta Brainwave Training," *Medical Psychotherapy* 3 (1990), 37-55, and Eugene G. Peniston and Paul J. Kulkosky, "Alpha-Theta Brainwave Training and Beta-Endorphin Levels in Alcoholics," *Alcoholism: Clinical and Experimental Research* 13 (1989), 271-79.

126 For a review and practical information about therapeutic touch, see Dolores Krieger, *The Therapeutic Touch: How to Use Your Hands to Help or to Heal* (Englewood Cliffs, N.J.: Prentice-Hall, 1979).

126 For popular articles see Elizabeth Stark, "Healing Hands," *Psychology Today* (1989), 29-30, and Jane E. Brody, "Laying On of Hands Gains New Respect," *New York Times*, March 26, 1985, 17, 20.

127 For articles by Janet Quinn, who has conducted research on therapeutic touch, see Quinn, "An Investigation of the Effects of Therapeutic Touch Done without Physical Contact on State of Anxiety of Hospitalized Cardiovascular Patients" Ph.D. dissertation, New York University, 1982, and Quinn, "Therapeutic Touch: The Empowerment of Love," *New Realities* (1987), 21-26.

128 The study by Dr. David Spiegel and associates of breast cancer patients can be found in D. Spiegel, J. R. Bloom, H. C. Kraemer, E. Gottheil, "Effect of Psychosocial Treatment on Survival of Patients with Metastatic Breast Cancer," *Lancet* (1989), 888-91.

128 The study on self-disclosure and immune function is reported by J. W. Pennebaker, J. K. Kiecolt-Glaser, and R. Glaser, "Disclosure of Traumas and Immune Function: Health Implications for Psychotherapy," *Journal of Consulting and Clinical Psychology* 56 (1988), 239-45, cited in Janice K. Kiecolt-Glaser and Ronald Glaser, "Mind and Immunity," Daniel Goleman and Joel Gurin, eds., *Mind/Body Medicine: How to Use Your Mind for Better Health* (Yonkers, N.Y.: Consumer Reports Books, 1993), 52-53, and E. J. Murray, A. D. Lamnin, and C. S. Carver, "Emotional Expression in Written Essays and Psychotherapy," *Journal of Social and Clinical Psychology* 8

Eighty-three-year-old Mildred Gianfagna is "cancer prone" — several of her relatives have died of breast cancer, and she has a benign lump under her arm that doctors check once a year. This page: *Still Life* (top) and *Floral* (bottom). Opposite page: *Still Life.*

Cartoons by Lisa Morrongiello were drawn in reaction to her illness and its treatments and medications.

(1989), 414-29.

129 D. Ornish, S. E. Brown, L. W. Scherwitz, et al. "Can Lifestyle Changes Reverse Coronary Heart Disease? The Lifestyle Heart Trial," *Lancet* 336 (July 21, 1990), 129-133. See also Dean Ornish, *Dr. Dean Ornish's Program for Reversing Heart Disease* (New York: Random House 1990), and Sharon R. Bard, "Healing the Heart: An Interview with Dean Ornish, MD," *Noetic Sciences Review* (Winter 1991), 13.

130 All material is from videotaped interviews from *The Heart of Healing* TBS television series.

133 Information about the First Nations People, the Stanford Arthritis Program, and the interaction between the arthritis program and Dr. Albert Bandura is from videotaped interviews in Port Alberni, British Columbia, and with Kate Lorig, Albert Bandura, and Halstead Holman from *The Heart of Healing* TBS television series.

135 Results of the experiments conducted with people who were terrified of snakes is reported in Sue A. Widenfeld, Ann O'Leary, Albert Bandura et al., "Impact of Perceived Self-Efficacy in Coping with Stressors on Components of the Immune System," *Journal of Personality and Social Psychology* 59 (1990), 1082-94, and in Ann O'Leary, "Self-Efficacy and Health," *Behavior Therapy* 23 (1985), 437-51. Additional information about snake phobia work is from videotaped interviews with O'Leary and Bandura from *The Heart of Healing* TBS television series.

136 Articles published about self-efficacy and the care of arthritis are Halstead Holman and Kate Lorig, "Perceived Self-Efficacy in Self-Management of Chronic Disease," in Ralf Schwarzer, ed., *Self-Efficacy: Thought Control of Action* (New York: Hemisphere Publications, 1992), 305-23; Kate Lorig and Virginia Gonzalez, "The Integration of Theory with Practice: A 12-Year Case Study," *Health Education Quarterly* 19 (1992), 355-368; Kate Lorig and James F. Fries, T*he Arthritis Helpbook: A Tested Self-Management Program for Coping with Your Arthritis* (Palo Alto, Calif.: Addison-Wesley, 1990).

134 Kristy Poindexter and her music therapist Joan Avanzino were videotaped for *The Heart of Healing* TBS television series.

134 Avram Goldstein, "Thrills in Response to Music and Other Stimuli," *Physiological Psychology* 8 (1980), 126-29; Robert E. Ornstein and David S. Sobel, "Getting a Dose of Musical Medicine. (Music Improves Health)," *Prevention* 41 (1989), 94-97.

134 The experiment at Rainbow Children's Hospital was conducted by Dr. Deforia Lane. See Deforia Lane, "Music Therapy: A Gift beyond Measure," *Oncology Nursing Forum* 19 (1992), 863-67, and *Journal of Oncology Management* 2 (1993), 42-46. Additional studies are reported by David M. Mazie, "Music's Surprising Power to Heal," *Reader's Digest* (1992); Anne H. Rosenfeld, "Music, the Beautiful Disturber; Whether It's Bach, Beatles, 'The Boss,' Blues or Ballads, Chances Are That Music Speaks to Your Emotions and It's No Accident," *Psychology Today* 19 (1985), 48-55.

134 Information about Oliver Sacks is in Teri Randall, "Music Not

Only Has Charms to Soothe, But Also to Aid Elderly in Coping with Various Disabilities," *Journal of the American Medical Association* 266 (September 11, 1991), 1323.

Chapter Six—Living and Healing

Page 141 The study of babies' recognition of their mothers' voices was performed by Anthony DeCasper and Melanie Spence and is reported along with other studies of voice recognition in fetuses in William Poole, "The First 9 Months of School," *Hippocrates* (July/August 1987), 68-73. Papers published on fetal voice recognition include: A. DeCasper and W. Fifer, "Of Human Bonding: Newborns Prefer Their Mothers' Voices," *Science* 208 (1980), 1174-76; A. DeCasper and M. Spence, "Prenatal Maternal Speech Influences Human Newborn Auditory Preferences," paper presented in 1982 at the Third Biennial International Conference on Infant Studies, Austin, Texas; R. K. Panneton, "Prenatal Auditory Experiences with Melodies: Effects on Post-Natal Auditory Preferences in Human Newborns," *Dissertation Abstracts* B (1985), 3984; and David B. Chamberlain, "Babies Are Not What We Thought: Call for a New Paradigm," *International Journal of Prenatal and Perinatal Studies* 4 (1992), 1-17.

141 The study that compared the activity of fetuses whose mothers were awaiting ultrasound with those whose mothers were awaiting ultrasound and amniocentesis is reported by N. Rossi, P. Avveduti, P. Rizzo, and R. Lorusso, "Maternal Stress and Fetal Motor Behavior: A Preliminary Report," *Journal of Developmental and Behavioral Pediatrics* 11 (1989), 190-94.

141 The effect of earthquakes on fetuses is reported by A. Ianniruberto and E. Tajani, "Ultrasonographic Study of Fetal Movements," *Seminars in Perinatology* 5 (1981), 175-81.

141 The research on the effect of maternal depression on the fetus is reported by B. Zuckerman, H. Bauchner, S. Parker, and H. Cabral, "Maternal Depressive Symptoms during Pregnancy, and Newborn Irritability," *Journal of Developmental and Behavioral Pediatrics* 11 (1990), 190-94, cited in Chamberlain, "Babies Are Not What We Thought," 7.

141 Research at the Minnesota Preschool Project is reported by Bruce Bower, "Caution: Emotions at Play," *Science News* 127 (April 27, 1985), 266-67. The Minnesota project is described in Izard, Kagan, and Zajonc, eds., *Emotions, Cognition and Behavior* (London: Cambridge University Press, 1984). The research is published in a number of papers, including B. Renken, B. Egeland, D. Marvinney et al., "Early Childhood Antecedents of Aggression and Passive-Withdrawal in Early Elementary School," *Journal of Personality* 57 (1989), 257-81, R. Kestenbaum, E. A. Farber, and L. A Sroufe, "Individual Differences in Empathy among Preschoolers: Relation to Attachment History," *New Directions in Child Development* (1989), 51-64; and M. Troy and L. A. Sroufe, "Victimization among Preschoolers: Role of Attachment Relationship History," *Journal of the American Academy of Child and Adolescent Psychiatry* 26 (1987), 166-72.

141 Erik Erikson, *Childhood and Society* (New York: Norton, 1963).

142 Elizabeth Hallett and Karen Ehrlich, *Midwife Means "With Woman"* (California Association of Midwives, Midwives' Awareness Project, 1991), 18; Marsden G. Wagner, "Infant Mortality in Europe: Implications for the United States: Statement to the National Commission to Prevent Infant Mortality," *Journal of Public Health Policy* 9 (1988), 75-78; and Judith P. Rooks, Norman L. Weatherby, Eunice K. M. Ernst et al., "Outcomes of Care in Birth Centers: The National Birth Center Study," *New England Journal of Medicine* 321 (December 28, 1989), 1804-11.

143 The story about Holy Roman Emperor Frederick II is in Peter B. Neubauer and Alexander Neubauer, "The Individual 'at Risk' in the Environment," *Mothering* (1992), 40-44, which is excerpted from Peter B. Neubauer and Alexander Neubauer, *Nature's Thumbprint: The New Genetics of Personality* (Palo Alto, Calif.: Addison-Wesley, 1990).

143 Information about the effect of placing babies evacuated from London in World War II in impersonal nurseries is found in Redford Williams, *The Trusting Heart* (New York: Times Books, 1989), 112.

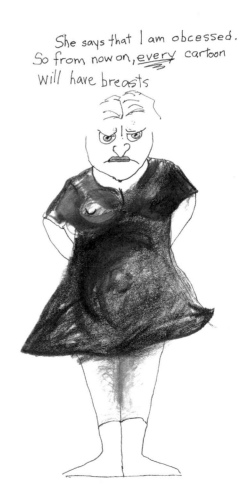

She says that I am obcessed. So from now on, _every_ cartoon will have breasts

143 The study of growth in rat pups separated from their mothers and preterm neonates is reported in S. M. Schanberg and T. M. Field, "Sensory Deprivation Stress and Supplemented Stimulation in the Rat Pup and Preterm Human Neonate," *Child Development* 58, 1431-47.

143 The research on the effects of stroking on premature infants is reported in T. M. Field, S. M. Schanberg, P. Scafidi et al., "Tactile/Kinesthetic Stimulation Effects on Preterm Neonates," *Pediatrics* 77 (1986), 654-58.

144 Michael T. Longaker and N. Scott Adzick, "The Biology of Fetal Wound Healing: A Review," *Plastic and Reconstructive Surgery* (April 1991), 788-98; H. Peter Lorenz, Michael T. Longaker, Luke A. Perkocha et al., "Scarless Wound Repair: A Human Fetal Skin Model," *Development* 114 (1992), 253-59; and N. Scott Adzick and Michael T. Longaker, "Scarless Fetal Healing: Therapeutic Implications," *Annals of Surgery* 215 (1992), 3-7.

145 Research on the effects of isolation on the brain development of rats is reported in M. C. Diamond, "Anatomical Brain Changes Induced by Environment," in L. Petrinovich and J. L. McGaugh, eds., *Knowing, Thinking and Believing* (New York: Plenum), 215-41, and in J. R. Connor and M. C. Diamond, "A Comparison of Dendritic Spine Number and Type on Pyramidal Neurons of the Visual Cortex of Old Adult Rats from Social or Isolated Environments," *Journal of Comparative Neurology* 210 (1982), 99-106.

145 Research from McGill and Stanford universities is reported in M. J. Meaney, D. H. Aitken, C. van Berkel et al., "Effect of Neonatal Handling on Age-Related Impairments Associated with the Hippocampus," *Science* 239 (February 12, 1988), 766-68. This study is cited in Williams, *The Trusting Heart*, 113. Subsequent research has been reported in a number of papers, including M. J. Meaney, J. B. Mitchell, D. H. Aitken et al., "The Effects of Neonatal Handling on the Development of the Adrenocortical Response to Stress: Implications for Neuropathology and Cognitive Deficits in Later Life," *Psychoneuroendocrinology* 16 (1991), 85-103.

145 Natalie Angier, "The Purpose of Playful Frolics: Training for Adulthood," *New York Times*, October 20, 1992, B5, and Jane E. Brody, "Personal Health: Prep Courses for Life: Dolls, Stickball, and Marbles," *New York Times*, October 21, 1992, B7.

145 Telephone interview with Carl E. Thoresen; C. E. Thoresen, "Type A and Teenagers," in R. Lerner, A. C. Petersen, and J. Brooks, eds., *Encyclopedia of Adolescence* (New York: Garland, 1990); C. E. Thoresen and J. Pattillo, "Exploring the Type A Behavior Pattern in Children and Adolescents," in B. K. Houston and C. R. Snyder, eds., *Type A Behavior: Research and Intervention* (New York: Wiley, 1988), 98-145; and Melinda Sacks, "Childhood in the Fast Lane," *Palo Alto Weekly*, September 5, 1990.

146 Lynn Payer, *Medicine and Culture* (New York: Penguin Books, 1988), and Lynn Payer, "Borderline Cases: How Medical Practice Reflects National Culture," *Sciences* (July-August 1990), 39-42.

148 The occurrence of sudden cardiac death was studied in 3,983 men, and it was found that an excess number occurred on Mondays. Among the men who had had heart disease, the deaths occurred more uniformly throughout the week. This study is reported in S. W. Rabkin, F. A. Mathewson, and R. B. Tate, "Chronobiology of Cardiac Sudden Death in Men," *Journal of the American Medical Association* 244 (September 19, 1980), 1357-58. The occurrence of sudden cardiac death in the morning, especially in the first three hours after awakening, is reported in a number of studies by James E. Muller and colleagues, who have noted that physiological measures, such as platelet aggregation, also increased in the morning. Papers on the subject include J. E. Muller, P. L. Ludmer, S. N. Willich et al., "Circadian Variation in the Frequency of Sudden Cardiac Death," *Circulation* 75 (1987), 131-38; J. E. Muller, "Morning Increase of Onset of Myocardial Infarction: Implications Concerning Triggering Events," *Cardiology* 76 (1989), 96-104; and J. E. Muller, G. H. Tofler, and E. Edelman, "Probable Triggers of Onset of Acute Myocardial Infarction," *Clinical Cardiology* 12 (1989), 473-75. These studies are cited in Larry Dossey, "Black Monday," *New Age Journal* (November/December 1991), 36-37, 99-100.

148 The 1990 survey of mental depression in one thousand families was presented at the annual meeting of the American Association for the Advancement of Science in February 1993 by Catherine E. Ross, a sociologist at the University of Illinois and is reported by Charles Petit, "Stay-at-Home Moms Ranked among the Most Depressed," *San Francisco Chronicle*, February 15, 1993, A3.

150 All information about the Apostolics and the Festival of Iemanja is from *The Heart of Healing* TBS television series.

152 The study in which students were shown a film about Mother Teresa is reported in J. Z. Borysenko, "Healing Motives: An Interview with David C. McClelland," *Advances* 2 (1985), 35-36.

152 L. F. Berkman and S. L. Syme, "Social Networks, Host Resistance and Mortality: A Nine-Year Follow-up Study of Alameda County Residents," *American Journal of Epidemiology* 109 (1979), 186-204.

152 The study of 2,800 elderly people was reported in E. L. Idler and S. V. Kasl, "Religion, Disability, Depression and the Timing of Death," *American Journal of Sociology* 97 (1992), 1052-79, and E. L. Idler, "Religious Involvement and the Health of the Elderly: Some Hypotheses and an Initial Test," *Social Forces* 66 (1987), 226-38. See also G. W. Comstock and K. B. Partridge, "Church Attendance and Health," *Journal of Chronic Diseases* 25 (1972), 665-72.

152 The review of two hundred studies of religion and mental health is reported by John Gartner, Dave B. Larson, and George D. Allen, "Religious Commitment and Mental Health: A Review of the Empirical Literature," *Journal of Psychology and Theology* 19 (1991), 6-25.

152 Randolph C. Byrd, "Positive Therapeutic Effects of Intercessory Prayer in a Coronary Care Unit Population," *Southern Medical*

Journal 81 (1988), 826-29.

152 Interview with George Solomon, from *The Heart of Healing* TBS television series, and Henry Dreher, "The Healthy Elderly and Long-Term Survivors of AIDS: Psychoimmune Connections," *Advances* 5 (1988), 6-12.

154 Norman Cousins, *Anatomy of an Illness as Perceived by the Patient* (New York: Norton, 1979), 71-75.

154 Telephone and videotaped interview with Joan Borysenko, from *The Heart of Healing* TBS television series.

155 All information about the Starcross Community is from videotaped interviews with community members from *The Heart of Healing* TBS television series.

158 Health-care statistics are from Institute for Health Policy Studies, University of California, San Francisco, Philip R. Lee, director, and Leonard A. Sagan, *The Health of Nations* (New York: Basic Books, 1987), 64.

159 Stanley Joel Reiser, "The Era of the Patient: Using the Experience of Illness in Shaping the Missions of Health Care," *Journal of the American Medical Association* 269 (February 24, 1993), 1012-17.

159 Debra Roter and Judith Hall, "Improving Psychosocial Problem Address in Primary Care: Is It Possible and What Difference Does It Make?" paper presented at the International Consensus Conference on Doctor-Patient Communication, November 14-16, 1991, Toronto, Canada; Debra L. Roter and Judith A. Hall, "Studies of Doctor-Patient Interaction," *Annual Review of Public Health* 10 (1989), 163-80. See also Daniel Goleman, "Doctors Find Comfort Is a Potent Medicine," *New York Times*, November 26, 1991, B8.

159 Results of study with elderly hip fracture patients is reported in J. J. Strain, "Psychotherapy and Medical Conditions," in Daniel Goleman and Joel Gurin, eds., *Mind/Body Medicine* (Yonkers, N.Y.: Consumer Reports Books, 1993), 367-83, and J. J. Strain, J. S. Lyons, J. S. Hammer et al., "Cost Offset from a Psychiatric Consultation-Liaison Intervention with Elderly Hip Fracture Patients," *American Journal of Psychiatry* 148 (1991), 44-49.

160 Diana B. Dutton, Worse *Than the Disease: Pitfalls of Medical Progress* (New York: Cambridge University Press, 1988), 4, 115-26, 304.

161 David M. Eisenberg, Ronald C. Kessler, Cindy Foster et al., "Unconventional Medicine in the United States: Prevalence, Costs and Patterns of U. S.," *New England Journal of Medicine* 328 (January 28, 1993), 246-252, and Edward W. Campion, "Why Unconventional Medicine?" *New England Journal of Medicine* 328 (January 28, 1993), 282-83.

162 Diana B. Dutton, "Poorer and Sicker: Legacies of the 1980s, Lessons for the 1990s," in S. Matteo, ed., *American Women in the Nineties: Today's Critical Issues* (Boston: Northeastern University Press, 1993), 108, 117.

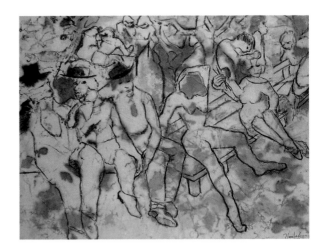

Three Hats in the Park (above) and *The Narcissist* (below) are by Norma Jabin, who beat the odds in 1979 when she was given only a 50 percent chance of surviving surgery for her breast cancer.

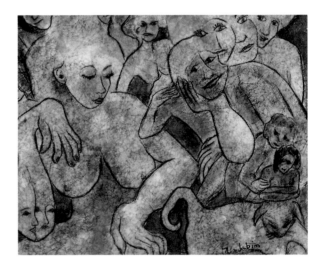

Achterberg, Jean. *Imagery and Healing: Shamanism and Modern Medicine*. Boston: New Science Library, 1985.

Achterberg, Jean, and G. Frank Lawlis. *Imagery and Disease*. Champaign, Ill.: Institute for Personality and Ability Testing, 1984.

Ader, Robert, ed. *Psychoneuroimmunology*. New York: Academic Press, 1981.

Anscombe , Elizabeth, and Peter Thomas Geach. *Philosophical Writings: Descartes*. London: Thomas Nelson and Sons, 1971.

Arehart-Treichel, Joan. *Biotypes: The Critical Link between Your Personality and Your Health*. New York: Times Books, 1980.

Beinfield, Harriet, and Efrem Korngold. *Between Heaven and Earth: A Guide to Chinese Medicine*. New York: Ballantine Books, 1991.

Benson, Herbert. *The Relaxation Response*. New York: Morrow, 1975.

Bloom, Floyd E., Arlyne Laxerson, and Laura Hofstadter. *Brain, Mind and Behavior*. New York: Freeman, 1985.

Bowlby, John. *Attachment and Loss*. Vols. 1-3. New York: Basic Books, 1969.

Boyd, William. *Spontaneous Regression of Cancer*. Springfield, Ill.: Charles C. Thomas, 1966.

Cannon, Walter. *The Wisdom of the Body*. New York: Norton, 1939.

Cleckley, Hervey, and Corbett Thigpen. *The Three Faces of Eve*. New York: McGraw-Hill, 1957.

Cohen, Sheldon, and S. Leonard Syme, eds. *Social Support and Health*. New York: Academic Press, 1985.

Cousins, Norman. *Anatomy of an Illness as Perceived by the Patient*. New York: Norton, 1979.

– – – . *Head First: The Biology of Hope and the Healing Power of the Human Spirit*. New York: Penguin Books, 1989.

– – – . *Human Options: An Autobiographical Notebook*. New York: Norton, 1981.

Dienstfrey, Harris. *Where the Mind Meets the Body*. New York: HarperCollins, 1991.

Dutton, Diana B. *Worse Than the Disease: Pitfalls of Medical Progress*. New York: Cambridge University Press, 1988.

Epstein, Alice Hopper. *Mind, Fantasy and Healing*. New York: Delacorte Press, 1989.

Erikson, Erik. *Childhood and Society*. New York: Norton, 1963.

Frank, Jerome. *Persuasion and Healing: A Comparative Study of Psychotherapy*. Baltimore: Johns Hopkins University Press, 1973.

Frey, William H., II. *Crying: The Mystery of Tears*. New York: Harper and Row, 1985.

Friedman, Meyer. *Treating Type A Behavior and Your Heart*. New York: Ballantine Books, 1984.

Goleman, Daniel, and Joel Gurin, eds. *Mind/Body Medicine: How to Use Your Mind for Better Health*. Yonkers, N.Y.: Consumer Reports Books, 1993.

Hilgard, Ernest, and Hilgard, Josephine. *Personality and Hypnosis: A Study of Imaginative Involvement*. Chicago: University of Chicago Press, 1979.

Houston, B. Kent, and Charles R. Snyder, eds. *Type A Behavior: Research and Intervention*. New York: Wiley, 1988.

Izard, Carroll E., Jerome Kagan, and Michael Zajonc, eds., *Emotions, Cognition and Behavior*. London: Cambridge University Press, 1984.

Justice, Blair. *Who Gets Sick*. Los Angeles: Jeremy P. Tarcher, 1988.

Kaptchuk, Ted J. *The Web That Has No Weaver: Understanding Chinese Medicine*. New York: Congdon and Weed, 1983.

Kaptchuk, Ted, and Michael Croucher. *The Healing Arts*. New York: Summit Books, 1987.

Katz, Richard. *Boiling Energy*. Boston: Harvard University Press, 1982.

Keyes, Daniel. *The Minds of Billy Milligan*. New York: Random House, 1981.

Krieger, Dolores. *The Therapeutic Touch: How to Use Your Hands to Help or to Heal*. Englewood Cliffs, N.J.: Prentice-Hall, 1979.

Lebra, Takie S., and William P. Lebra, eds. *Japanese Culture and Behavior*. Honolulu: Unversity Press of Hawaii, 1974.

Lee, Philip R., and Leonard A. Sagan. *The Health of Nations*. New York: Basic Books, 1987.

Locke, Steven, and Douglas Colligan. *The Healer Within*. New York: E. P. Dutton, 1986.

Lorig, Kate, and James F. Fries. *The Arthritis Helpbook: A Tested Self-Management Program for Coping with Your Arthritis*. Palo Alto, Calif.: Addison-Wesley, 1990.

Lyons, Albert S., and R. Joseph Petrucelli. *Medicine: An Illustrated History*. New York: Abradale Press, 1987.

MacLean, Paul. *A Truine Concept of the Brain and Behavior*. Toronto: University of Toronto Press, 1973.

Maddi, Salvatore R., and Suzanne C. Kobasa. *The Hardy Executive: Health under Stress*. Homewood, Ill.: Dow Jones-Irwin, 1984.

Matteo, Sherri, ed. *American Women in the Nineties: Today's Critical Issues*. Boston: Northeastern University Press, 1993.

Murphy, Michael. *The Future of the Body*. Los Angeles: Jeremy P. Tarcher, 1992.

Myers, Frederick W. *Human Personality and Its Survival of Bodily Death*. Vols. 1 and 2. Salem, N.H.: Ayre, 1975.

Neubauer, Peter B., and Alexander Neubauer. *Nature's Thumbprint: The New Genetics of Personality*. Palo Alto, Calif.: Addison-Wesley, 1990.

Nuland, Sherwin B. *Doctors: The Biography of Medicine*. New York: Knopf, 1988.

O'Regan, Brendan, and Caryle Hirshberg. *Spontaneous Remission — An Annotated Bibliography*. Sausalito, Calif.: Institute of Noetic Sciences, 1993.

Ornish, Dean. *Dr. Dean Ornish's Program for Reversing Heart Disease*. New York: Random House 1990.

Ornstein, Robert, and David Sobel. *The Healing Brain*. New York: Simon and Schuster, 1987.

Ornstein, Robert, and Richard F. Thompson. *The Amazing Brain*. Boston: Houghton Mifflin, 1984.

Payer, Lynn. *Medicine and Culture*. New York: Penguin Books, 1988.

Petrinovich, Lewis, and James L. McGaugh, eds. *Knowing, Thinking and Believing*. New York: Plenum, 1976.

Platonov, K. *The Word as a Psychological and Therapeutic Factor*. Moscow: Foreign Language Publishing House, 1959.

Podmore, Frank. *From Mesmer to Christian Science*. New York: University Books, 1963.

Price, Virginia A. *Type A Behavior Pattern: A Model for Research and Practice*. New York: Academic Press, 1982.

Rogo, D. Scott. *Miracles: A Parascientific Inquiry into Wondrous Phenomena*. New York: Dial Press, 1982.

Scherer, Klaus R., and Paul Ekman, eds. *Approaches to Emotion*. Hillsdale, N.J.: Lawrence Erlbaum, 1984.

Schindler, Lydia W. *Understanding the Immune System*. Bethesda, Md.: National Institutes of Health, 1991.

Schreiber, Flora Rheta. *Sybil*. New York: Warner Books, 1974.

Schwarzer, Ralf, ed. *Self-Efficacy: Thought Control of Action*. New York: Hemisphere Publications, 1992.

Seligman, Martin E. P. *Learned Optimism*. New York: Simon and Schuster, 1990.

Selye, Hans. *The Physiology and Pathology of Exposure to Stress*. Montreal: Acta, 1975.

Sheikh, Anees A., ed. *Imagination and Healing*. Amityville, N.Y.: Baywood Publishing, 1984.

Simonton, O. Carl, Stephanie Matthews-Simonton, and James Creighton. *Getting Well Again*. New York: Bantam Books, 1981.

Stoyva, Johann, et al., eds. *Biofeedback and Self-Control, 1977/78*. Chicago: Aldine, 1978.

Temoshok, Lydia, and Henry Dreher. *The Type C Connection: The Behavioral Links to Cancer and Your Health*. New York: Random House, 1992.

Thomas, Lewis. *The Medusa and the Snail*. New York: Viking, 1979.

Weatherhead, Leslie D. *Psychology, Religion and Healing*. Nashville: Abington Press, 1952.

Weil, Andrew. *Health and Healing*. Boston: Houghton Mifflin, 1988.

White, Leonard, Bernard Tursky, and Gary E. Schwartz. *Placebo: Theory, Research and Mechanisms*. New York: Guilford Press, 1985.

Williams, Redford. *The Trusting Heart*. New York: Times Books, 1989.

INDEX

ART CREDITS